**strong,
calm
and free**

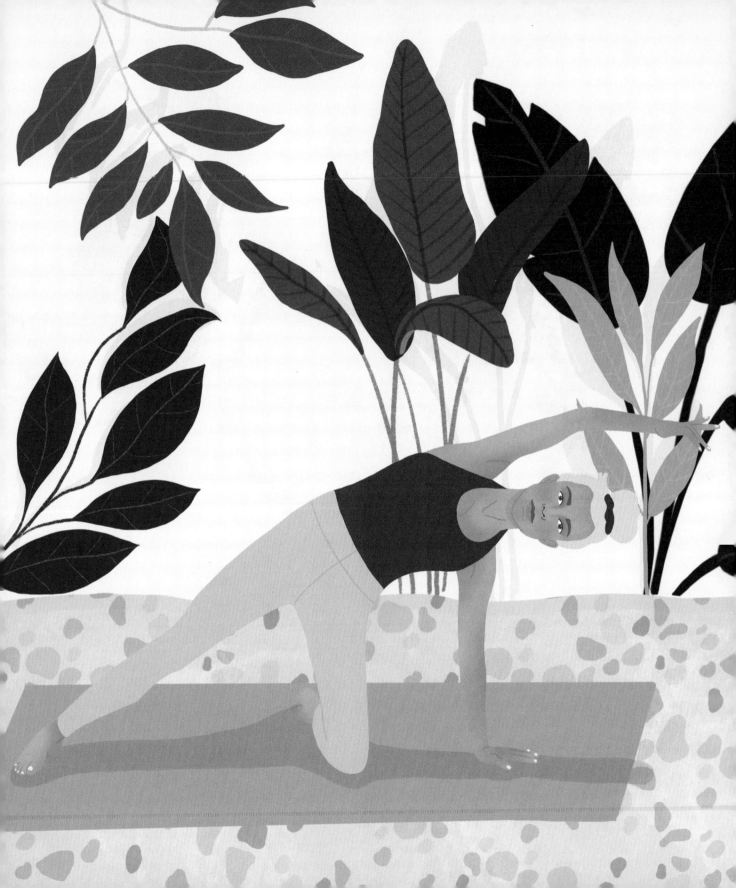

nicola jane hobbs

strong, calm and free

A MODERN GUIDE TO YOGA, MEDITATION AND MINDFUL LIVING

GREEN TREE
LONDON • OXFORD • NEW YORK • NEW DELHI • SYDNEY

GREEN TREE
Bloomsbury Publishing Plc
50 Bedford Square, London, WC1B 3DP, UK
29 Earlsfort Terrace, Dublin 2, Ireland

BLOOMSBURY, GREEN TREE and the
Green Tree logo are trademarks of
Bloomsbury Publishing Plc

First published in Great Britain 2021

A catalogue record for this book is
available from the British Library

Library of Congress Cataloguing-in-
Publication data has been applied for

ISBN: PB: 978-14729-7977-3;
eBook: 978-14729-7976-6;
ePdf: 978-14729-7975-9

10 9 8 7 6 5 4 3 2

Design by Austin Taylor

Printed in China by
RRD Asia Printing Solutions Limited

Bloomsbury Publishing Plc makes every
effort to ensure that the papers used in
the manufacture of our books are natural,
recyclable products made from wood grown
in well-managed forests. Our manufacturing
processes conform to the environmental
regulations of the country of origin.

To find out more about our authors and
books visit www.bloomsbury.com and
sign up for our newsletters

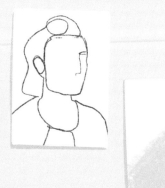

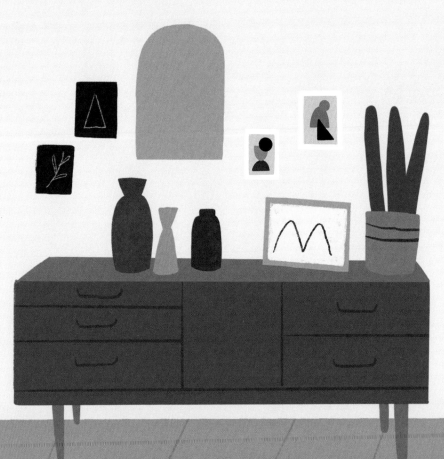

Contents

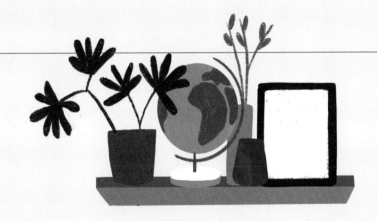

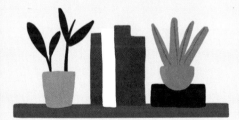

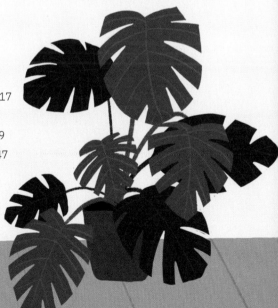

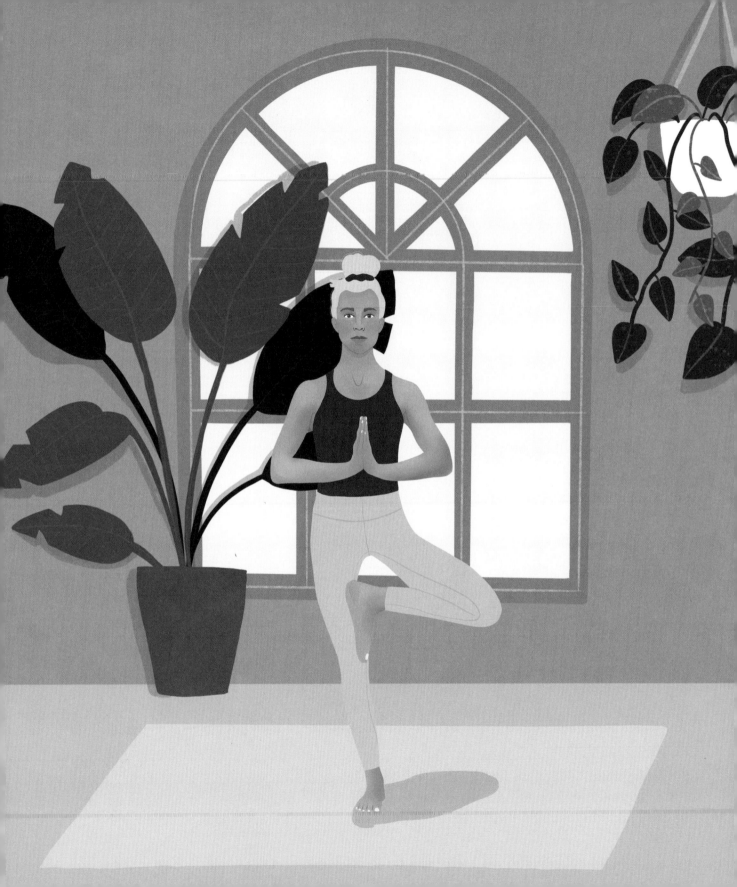

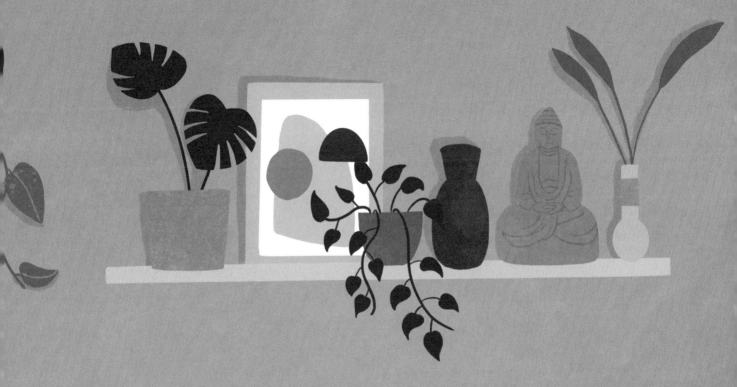

Introduction

The Gift of Yoga

NOT LONG AFTER MY 18TH BIRTHDAY, I found myself sitting cross-legged on a yoga mat at the back of a local yoga studio. The smoky smell – a potent blend that reminded me of Christmas spices – was slowly diffusing around the room and there was gentle, uplifting music playing with lyrics in a language I didn't understand. I had never practised yoga before. I thought meditation was for monks. And mindfulness was yet to make it to the mainstream. But I was finding the intense pressure and machine pace of modern life overwhelming and I was willing to try anything to take the edge off the ever-present anxiety that hummed beneath the surface of my life.

The yoga teacher instructed us to stand at the top of our mat and asked us to silently set a *sankalpa*, an intention for our practice: why had we come to class today? Who would we like to dedicate our practice to? How could we make our time on the mat sacred? I felt awkward. Uncomfortable. Vulnerable. In my mind, yoga was like aerobics or spinning – a workout, a way to get fit and let off steam. I wasn't interested in the spiritual stuff. But, by the end of the class, something deep within me had ever-so-slightly shifted – softened, opened, released – and, after years of feeling anxious, overwhelmed and exhausted, I felt different. I felt strong, calm and free. I glimpsed what it was like to be fully present, fully in my body instead of stuck in my head judging it from the

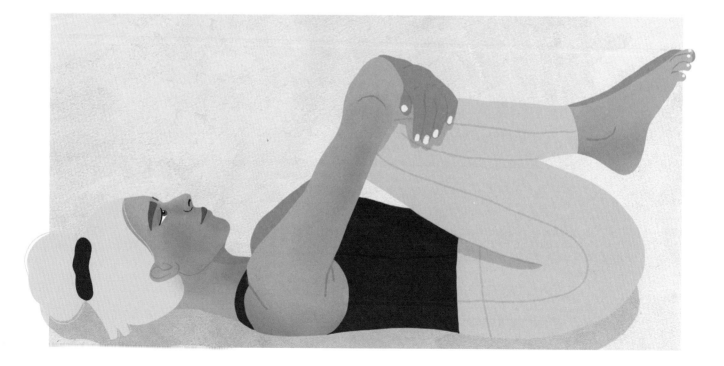

outside. And, for a brief moment, the coppery voice of my inner critic faded and I touched an inner peace that I had forgotten existed. It was as if I had spent my whole life holding my breath and now I could finally exhale.

I went back to class every week after that. Learning how to breathe again. Learning the poses and their funny Sanskrit names. Learning how to be in my body in a way that was nourishing and not destructive. Learning how to be present instead of always striving towards the next goal. Learning how to be strong. And how to surrender.

A couple of years later, I booked a flight to Thailand to train as a yoga and meditation teacher. And I've been sharing the gift of yoga ever since. Both my practice and teaching have changed a lot over the last decade. In the early days, the advanced poses – the fancy arm balances and extreme backbends – were the goal of my practice. But, over the years, I have discovered the poses are just the beginning, an entry point to a practice that will, if you let it, transform your entire life.

Most people come to yoga for the poses – and it is these poses that modern, fitness-based yoga largely focuses on – but they are just a tiny part of a deeper, richer, more beautiful journey that has been travelled for thousands of years as a path to health, happiness and wholeness. It is this wholeness that I would like to share in this book. Because, when you sense the sheer lavishness of the practice, you will begin to see how yoga is not a workout or a tool for self-improvement. Nor is it a way to relax before jumping back into the busyness of everyday life. It's not something you do once a week or whenever you have time. Instead, yoga is a practice that saturates your whole life. A practice in letting go, loving deeply and living fully. It is a compassionate, flowering adventure towards a more peaceful, joyful way of being in the world. It is a journey towards wholeness. Towards freedom. Towards becoming fully and completely who we are.

I have written this book for anyone who feels called to explore the universe of yoga – for those of you who are totally new to yoga or new to teaching yoga and also

Yoga is a practice that saturates your whole life. It is a compassionate, flowering adventure towards a more peaceful, joyful way of being in the world. Towards becoming fully and completely who we are.

for those of you who would like to deepen your practice and recommit to this spiritual adventure once more. Yoga is so immense, that, even after a decade of practising and teaching, I still see myself as a beginner. And I find myself beginning my yoga journey again and again, year after year, breath after breath – returning to the same pose over and over again, each time with a heart that is a little more open and a little less afraid.

The 18-year-old who first set foot on the yoga mat all those years ago was an anxious, ego-driven, achievement-orientated perfectionist, rushing through life and chasing after goals that didn't really matter to her in an attempt to prove she was good enough. If I could speak to her now, I would remind her to slow down and breathe deeply and listen inwardly for what her heart has to say. I would reassure her that her struggles can be the very source of her awakening – the very places where joy, wisdom and love can flourish. I would encourage her to keep practising, to keep returning to her yoga mat, to keep creating a sacred space where self-awareness and self-respect can blossom.

And this is what I would like to tell you too. Because through yoga we can find something we cannot find elsewhere. A peace, a beauty, a wholeness. This is why I wrote this book. Because, as a yoga and meditation teacher and holistic counsellor, I see how many people are struggling. I see how many people need a sacred space, an island of relief among the chaos of their lives to reconnect with their body, reclaim their power and remember their beauty.

This is the gift of yoga.

What is Yoga?

WE HAVE STONE-AGE NERVOUS SYSTEMS. We are born expecting a rich and sensuous relationship with ourselves, each other and the natural world. We are born with an innate longing for connection, for belonging, for wholeness. To become fully and completely who we are. Without self-doubt. Without holding back. Without hiding the parts of ourselves that are difficult to love. Yoga is the union of everything we must do to realise this wholeness.

This is the central premise of this book: we are whole, we are worthy and every single piece of us is sacred. And, with some simple practices, we can begin to realise this wholeness. To remember who we are beneath the masks we wear. To reconnect with why we are here and what is important. To know ourselves as more than a body and a brain but as the lifeforce that flows through all beings, the divine spark that shimmers and glitters in our heart and floods our whole being with aliveness. Because, when we meet ourselves unmasked for the first time – hiding beneath the layers of cultural conditioning and other people's opinions – we discover our beauty, our strength, our limitless love. And, once we realise this, we become available to the world – to share, to serve, to love – with a deep and beautiful trust in our body, our intuition and life itself.

Modern life means that many of us have become disconnected from this wholeness. We have forgotten who we are and why we are here. We feel lost and lonely – alienated from our body, isolated from community and cut off from nature. We experience health problems – acid reflux, anxiety, asthma, depression, irritable bowel syndrome, lower back pain and osteoporosis – because our lifestyles have become so disconnected from how humans are born to live. And many of us have forgotten what it feels like to be healthy and happy, to wake up each day with energy and excitement, to feel fully alive.

Yoga is a journey of remembering, reconnecting and reawakening. The word itself comes from the Sanskrit – the oldest language in India – root, *yuj*, meaning to 'yoke' or 'unite'. It is both a state of connection and a collection of techniques that together allow us to feel more connected to ourselves, each other and life; a tool to help us remember who we are. This journey of reconnection usually begins with the yoga poses themselves; with stepping on your yoga mat and breathing and moving in a way that makes you feel stronger and calmer, that frees you from regrets about the past and worries about the future and connects you with this breath, this body, this moment, right here, right now.

For most of us, when we begin yoga, this physical practice is all we are interested in. It is all we know. Modern postural yoga is often taught as a form of exercise – like running or CrossFit – and it has many of the same health benefits as working out (increased strength, improved flexibility, greater bone density, decreased blood pressure and a stronger immune system). But, in many ways, yoga is the opposite of working out. Whereas many types of exercise deplete the body, increase cortisol and produce lactic acid (often leaving you sore and exhausted), practising yoga reduces stress hormones, develops muscles in a balanced way to build both strength

Yoga is a journey of remembering, reconnecting and reawakening.

and flexibility, and has a soothing effect on the nervous system to cultivate energy, vitality and tranquillity.

Because *asanas* – yoga poses – often serve as the entry point, much of this book is dedicated to the physical practice of yoga: clear illustrations of each pose with detailed instructions to help you find your way back into your body and be present with whatever arises – tension, strength, stability, heat, release, pressure, grace, beauty, power – as well as simple sequences you can learn by heart so that you feel confident in your self-practice.

It took at least a year of going to yoga classes and practising the poses at home for me to begin exploring yoga off the mat: meditation, philosophy, scripture. My physical practice opened me to another way of seeing the world and another way of being in the world. One where I felt called to journey deeper in to myself and to allow my life to be changed by what I discovered. For this reason, I have shared many other branches of yoga in this book – all rooted in mindful living – and ways you can practise these in your daily life. This deeper journey might not be what you want or need right now, so, if you've come to yoga purely for a stronger core or looser hamstrings, then feel free to ignore the deeper spiritual aspects until you feel called to explore them further. The traditions of yoga are not meant to indoctrinate us but to inspire us. Take what you need and leave the rest behind.

> At its core, yoga is not religious, supernatural or otherworldly, but rooted in living a life that is ethical, compassionate and kind

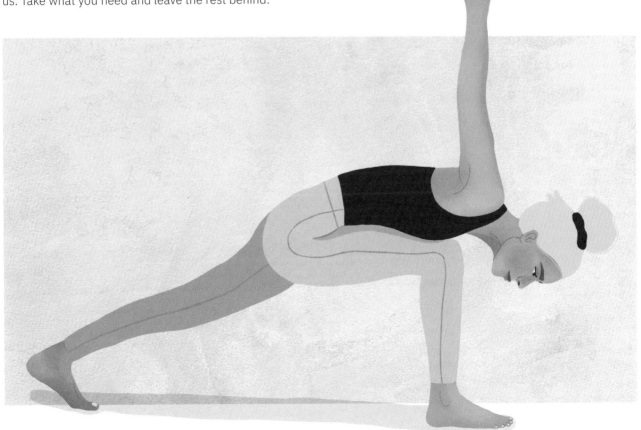

If you are interested in exploring yoga as a more holistic lifestyle practice – a way of being in the world – then I have attempted to share some of the essential ideas and practices in a way that is accessible and allows yoga to evolve for 21st-century living without losing its essence. If you are anything like me, you might find some of the more mystical words – such as 'god', 'divinity' and 'oneness' – challenging at first. Don't let semantics hold you back. Create your own definition of 'spirituality', decide what 'divine' means to you, get to know your personal 'god'. At its core, yoga is not religious, supernatural or otherworldly, but rooted in living a life that is ethical, compassionate and kind.

What you'll find in this book is not a definitive guide to the practice or philosophy of yoga (their sheer enormity means that it would be impossible to share in one book!), but my own interpretation based on my self-practice, my teaching and my work integrating the ancient wisdom of yoga with modern psychology. If you'd like to explore the scriptures and history of yoga at a deeper level, you'll find a list of recommended reading on page 188.

Before you begin, I would encourage you to contemplate what yoga means to you. What would you like to get out of your practice? And what you are willing to invest in it? This understanding will evolve over time, and, through the ten-week journey in Part Two of the book, your relationship with yoga will change and grow. Saying this, yoga is largely a journey of unlearning, of letting go of expectations and opening to our present experience, whatever that might be. In this way, before we begin our practice, it is helpful to unlearn what we think yoga *should* be: what the poses *should* look like, how many times we *should* get on our mat each week, when we *should* be able to touch our toes or balance on our head or do a handstand

Strong, Calm and Free

I called this book *Strong, Calm and Free* because that is what yoga has become for me – a journey to strength, peace and freedom. I refer to *strength* in the widest possible sense: a strong body that has been built through movement, rest and nourishment, a strong mind that allows you to make conscious choices in your life instead of being overpowered by the demands of the world and an inner strength that shines within you like the sun, offering others a light when they can't see. *Calmness* is about living with peace, patience and a quiet inner power. It's about realising you are the bright blue sky and not the passing clouds. The eye at the centre of every storm. The loving awareness that exists behind every fleeting thought, emotion and craving. Yoga is a journey into the depths of yourself. And, just like in the ocean, when waves are crashing down on the surface of your life, go deep enough and you will find stillness. *Freedom* means being free to feel the full force of our feelings without being overwhelmed by them. It means being free from attachment and addiction and the critical voice in your head that says you are unlovable or unworthy. It means to be free to choose the kind of life you want to live instead of being pushed and pulled around by automatic thoughts, harmful habits and other people's expectations. It means the freedom to be fully and fearlessly yourself. A verse from the *Yoga Sutras*, widely regarded as the authoritative text on yoga, captures freedom beautifully, 'We are not going to change the whole world, but we can change ourselves and feel free as birds.'

Yoga is deeply personal and profoundly universal. Yoga is a path to health, happiness and wholeness. Yoga is an inner journey. A journey home to ourselves. Yoga is opening a conversation with our body and our soul. Yoga is a way to see the world more clearly and love it more deeply. Yoga is welcoming every part of what it means to be human – the love and the loss, the dark and the light, the hurt and the healing. Yoga is paying attention. Yoga is listening. Yoga is connecting to your breath, your body, your feelings, your thoughts, whatever is going on between you and the Universe right now. Yoga is a way of living. One where you are no longer trapped in your head but fully present, fully connected to each moment. Yoga is a way to balance the mainstream messages of our culture. A reminder that there is nothing to prove and you are good enough just the way you are. Yoga is an opening. A deepening. A remembering of what it means to be human. A singing, dancing, loving, crying, feeling, breathing, hugging human. Yoga is a path to falling in love with the world and everything in it so you can make the most of these precious breaths we call life.

How to Use this Book

IT IS NOT SELF-INDULGENT or egotistical or silly to work on your inner life, to nurture your inner garden, to explore your inner world. In fact, if we are to experience inner peace, deep joy and true love, this inner work is essential. This book is a guide and invitation to begin this inner journey. It's main purpose is not to give you lots of information about yoga but to wake you up to the love and joy that is possible when you start practising it; to open you to a more loving, peaceful, joy-filled way of being in the world.

The book itself is divided into three sections: Part One intends to inspire you, Part Two is the practice itself – a ten-week journey of yoga, meditation and mindful living – and Part Three offers you extra sequences for grounding, calming and energising.

Part One introduces you to some of the key concepts of yoga, mindfulness and well-being that will enhance your practice. Yoga has a rich and beautiful history and this will help you get a feel for the transformative power that your practice can have on your life. It is written in an essay format, which means that you can read a few pages at a time without feeling like you need to get through the whole thing before you step on your mat and begin the yoga journey itself.

Our practice is where yoga comes alive instead of simply being a collection of abstract ideas, so the bulk of the book is made up of the ten-week journey, which includes discussions, sequences, meditations and mindful-living practices. This journey is designed to be travelled alongside the support of a yoga teacher at a studio or as a stand-alone self-practice that you can practise at home as a form of self-care. I have created the sequences so that you can learn them by heart and adapt them to fit in with whatever time you have. In this way, you will become your own teacher.

This book is not one of extremes. It is a middle path. Not one of juice fasts or silent retreats or yoga marathons in boiling-hot rooms, but of awareness, compassion and love.

This book is not one of extremes. It is a middle path. Not one of juice fasts or silent retreats or yoga marathons in boiling-hot rooms, but of awareness, compassion and love.

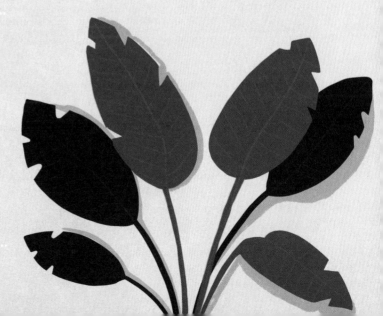

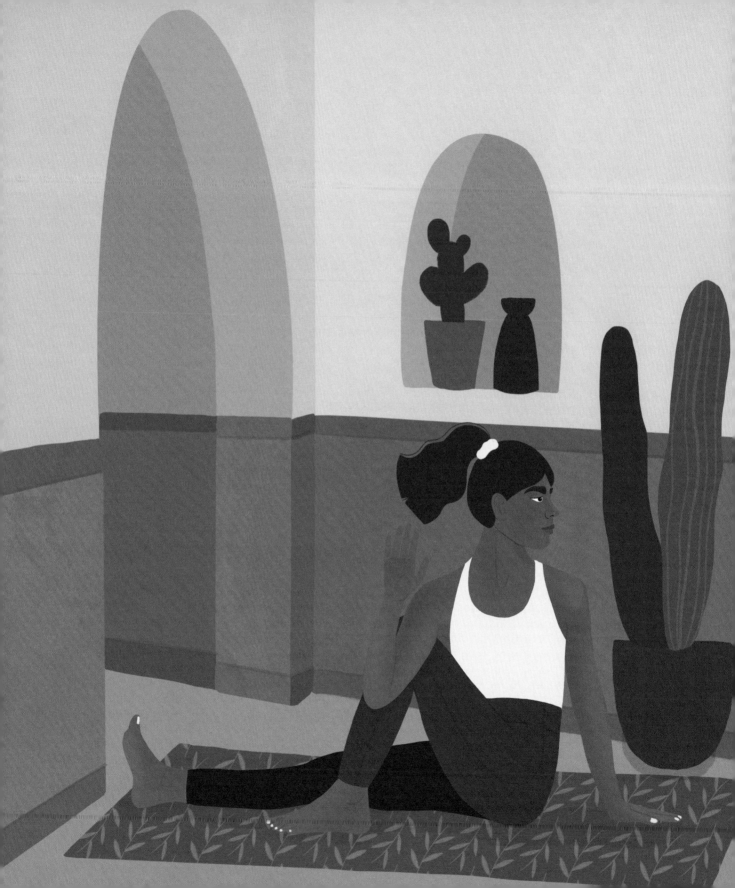

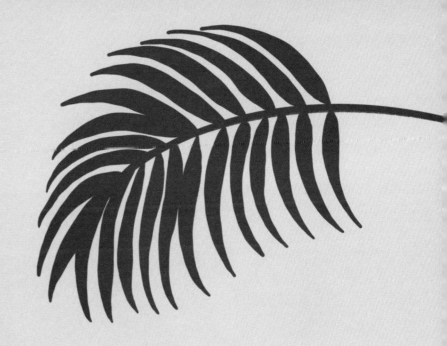

PART ONE

Wisdom

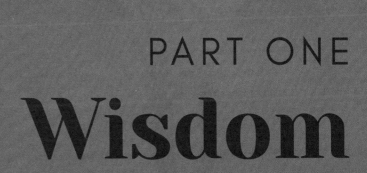

The Eight Limbs of Yoga

IN THE WEST, we have come to see yoga as the physical practice of poses, but the philosophy of yoga is a rich and beautiful thing that can open us to a deeper, calmer, more meaningful way of being alive. The trouble is, it can be overwhelming. There is so much of it, many of the words are in Sanskrit, and the concepts often feel so alien to our Western minds that we struggle to grasp them. But, at its essence, the philosophy of yoga gifts us two things: The true goal of yoga – to discover a state of health and wholeness that exists within each of us – and a practical path to follow so that we can free ourselves from suffering and dissatisfaction and experience this wholeness and aliveness for ourselves.

Having a basic understanding of yoga philosophy also gives us a much broader view of yoga and reminds us that yoga is so much bigger than the poses themselves. At different points in our life – illness, ageing, disability, fatigue, travel and during particularly hectic periods – we may not be able to get on our yoga mat for an intense physical practice. But, by weaving in other threads of yoga – meditation, breathwork, self-reflection, compassion and gratitude practices – we cultivate a deeper relationship with yoga that can transform our lives.

You learn yoga philosophy slowly – how to read it, how to understand it, and how to apply it to your life. I picked up many books on yoga philosophy when I first began my practice – the *Yoga Sutras*, the *Bhagavad Gita*, the *Upanishads* – and put them down after a page or two because I couldn't understand a word. Now when I read those texts, they touch my heart so deeply that I wonder how they never made sense before. This is how yoga works: a soft and gentle awakening that comes with practice and patience.

The eight limbs of yoga, sometimes called the eightfold path to freedom, is one of the most accessible elements of yoga philosophy that is applicable to modern life. It is a template for how to live with less stress and suffering and more joy and freedom, a series of guideposts to help us remember who we are, why we are here and the wholeness that exists within us.

You'll find each of the limbs woven into the ten-week journey in Part Two of the book. Don't worry too much if some of the limbs don't make sense yet. As your practice deepens, your understanding will too.

The first two limbs of yoga, the *yamas* and *niyamas*, are known as the ten pillars of mindful living or the ten pillars of wisdom. They give us guidelines for living an ethical life so we can live more peacefully and joyfully. The *yamas* consist of five ways to live in a more moral and meaningful way: non-harm, non-lying, non-stealing, non-grasping and non-excess. The second branch, the *niyamas*, are five daily practices that cultivate inner strength, confidence and happiness: self-discipline, unconditional acceptance, cleansing, self-study and self-surrender. You can read about these in more detail on page 22.

The yoga poses, known as *asanas*, make up the third branch of the eightfold path. The literal translation of *asana* is 'seat'. Traditionally, we use the physical postures to prepare the body to sit in meditation (tight muscles are distracting when you're trying to meditate!). Rather than forcing our body into advanced arm balances or aesthetically impressive backbends, the word *asana* reminds us to 'sit' in each posture, to find comfort in the pose – a balance between strength and softness – so we're not distracted by aches and pains or restless because we're pushing the body into positions it is simply not ready for. The paradoxical phrase 'effortless effort' beautifully captures this attitude to practising *asanas*. Having a regular *asana* practice also helps us to develop discipline and focus, as well as keeping the body healthy and strong, which, as Zen master Thich Nhat Hanh says, 'is an expression of gratitude to the whole cosmos'. We explore the physical practice more on page 48.

Breath is everything in yoga. Breathwork, known as *pranayama*, is the fourth branch of the eightfold path. The breath is a bridge between the mind and body, an anchor to the present moment, an ever-present tool that can bring us out of our head and into the only place life exists: now. There is an assortment of ancient breathing practices – some cleansing, some calming, some invigorating – and we'll explore many of them throughout our ten-week journey.

The fifth branch of yoga, *pratyahara*, literally means 'gaining mastery over external influences' and is often referred to as 'withdrawal of the senses'. We live in a consumeristic society full of sensory overload – loud noises, artificial lights, social media, advertising, caffeine – which keeps us distracted from looking within ourselves and finding out who we are and what we really need (play, intimacy, connection, nature, belonging) beneath the things society says we need (flawless faces, perfect bodies, high salaries, big houses, fancy cars, fast food). One of the best ways to practise *pratyahara* is to reduce the amount of stimulation we are bombarded with on a daily basis: turn off the radio when you're

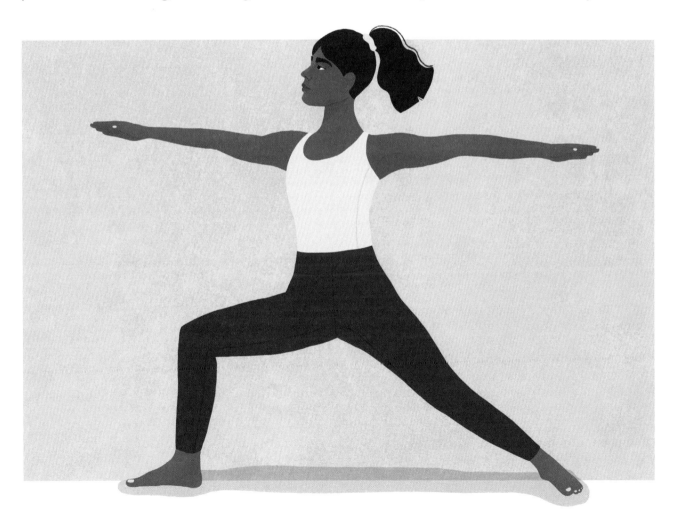

driving, put your phone away after seven o'clock, avoid watching violent movies, replace your weekend shopping spree with a long walk in the woods, or simply take a few minutes each day to sit with your eyes closed. *Pratyahara* provides us with a way to become conscious of any habits that may be harming our health so our cravings and urges no longer overpower us. Instead of walking past the bakery one minute and the next minute finding yourself halfway through a family-size bag of doughnuts (even though eating gluten gives you stomach ache), *pratyahara* provides us with a way to take a step back and objectively observe our cravings. This gives us the freedom to make choices that lead to greater health, happiness and wholeness rather than being pushed and pulled around by the bombardment of temptations and desires in the external world.

As we move further down the eightfold path, the focus shifts from the external world – mindful living through values such as non-violence, physical strength through poses and vitality through breathing practices – to the inner world and the cultivation of consciousness so we can live in a way that feels more authentic, more awake, more alive. *Dharana*, meaning 'concentration', is the sixth branch of yoga. Now that we have reduced distractions in the external world through *pratyahara*, *dharana* involves reducing the distractions of our inner world – the endless stream of thoughts that ripple through our mind and take us away from the present moment. We can learn to find this focus by concentrating on a single object – the breath, a mental image, the flickering flame of a candle – and, with practice, we will be able to hold our attention on this object for longer periods of time without our mind wandering to that email we need to send or that thing our colleague said to us yesterday or what we're going to have for dinner!

The seventh branch of yoga, *dhyana* – meditation – comes quite naturally from periods of concentration. The difference is that, while *dharana* involves effort, *dhyana* is effortless; a kind of defocusing while staying awake and aware. It is a both a practice of being with what is in the present moment – pain, fear, grief, joy, hope, anger, frustration – without judgement, and a state of being where you are completely yourself – no thoughts, no worries, no masks; a feeling of wholeness,

a sense of oneness. This state of deep concentration is what psychology calls 'flow state'. It is the experience of being 'in the zone' when we are so present and focused on what we are doing that everything else – including our usual mind chatter – melts away. This is the state athletes are in when they perform their best, writers are in when they are their most creative, businesspeople are in when they are most productive and all humans are in when they feel the most joy, the most meaning, the most alive. Sometimes, this state of *dhyana* can take a lifetime of practice to experience and other times we glimpse it at random moments in daily life when we are fully present, deeply relaxed and totally alive.

The final branch of yoga is *samadhi,* more commonly called 'enlightenment'. This can be seen as a caterpillar becoming a butterfly. A deep and beautiful transformation in the way we experience the world. In some traditions, reaching enlightenment – transcending the individual self and merging with the divine – is treated as a goal that is attainable to very few. But enlightenment can also be very human, very accessible and very ordinary. As Zen master Shunryu Suzuki said, 'There are, strictly speaking, no enlightened people, there is only enlightened activity.' In this way, instead of seeing enlightenment as some holier-than-thou state reserved for gurus and masters, enlightenment becomes a way of being in the world. One where we meet each moment with awareness and acceptance, replace automatic reactions with mindful responses, rooted in deep compassion, and breathe light and love into everything we do. In many ways, enlightenment is about bringing more light into the world; being a candle, a lamp, a lighthouse for those who are lost.

As you can see, the eightfold path is not some aggressive self-improvement project calling for grand action or harsh deprivation. All it asks of us is that we bring our kind and loving attention to our breath, our body, our mind, our intentions, our actions, our families, our communities and our planet. This is all that matters: that we begin here and now to practise and live with more awareness. This soft and gentle awareness is enough to transform our lives.

The Essence and Evolution of Yoga

I am a white, British woman teaching an ancient spiritual practice which originated in India thousands of years ago. Over the years, some of those who have come to me for teaching have told me they are 'only interested in the stretches' and studio owners have asked me not to include anything 'too spiritual' in my classes — without realising that yoga *is* a spiritual practice.

I have made many mistakes in the past, watering down my teaching in an attempt to make yoga more accessible in the West, not realising that this was misrepresenting the history, culture and purpose of yoga and stripping away its essence.

'The mind creates the abyss, the heart crosses it,' the Indian spiritual teacher Sri Nisargadatta Maharaj said. And, over the last few years I have been focusing on crossing the abyss, learning about the history and roots of yoga and acknowledging that much of what I teach originates from historically oppressed communities. There is still a lot I don't know and I am not the right person to write about the decolonisation of yoga but I am learning how important it is to create space in our yoga practice to reflect on, educate ourselves in and honour the ancient lineages we have the privilege of accessing.

Moving below the surface of our yoga practice by exploring and honouring its roots is a lifelong process, often revealing to us our privileges — social advantages we may have based on things such as race, sexual orientation, religion, socioeconomic status, language and ability. This can be heavy work and there will times in our life when we have greater emotional capacity to do it than others.

We can begin where we are: by learning, practising and living all eight limbs of yoga (*see* pp. 16–18) instead of just the poses, by reading ancient scriptures and spiritual books from different cultures and traditions (there is a list of recommended reading on page 188) and by exploring the meaning of any spiritual ornaments or symbols we might have around our home or on our clothes (for example, Buddha figurines, mandala paintings, the Aum symbol on a yoga top). We can also start asking ourselves the more difficult questions: *What parts of yoga am I leaving out and why? Does the yoga I practise promote peace for all? How might my practice be an opportunity to address injustice and inequality?*

I am learning that what many of us are looking for when we begin our yoga journey is the very thing modern Western yoga so often leaves behind: practices and rituals that nourish and empower us, that give us something greater than ourselves to connect with and belong to, that offer us something deeper and more meaningful than the shallow materialism of modern society.

If we open to it, if we are willing to go deeper than the physical, if we do our best to humbly honour the ancient yogic teachings, we can move into this sacred space of deep listening, loving awareness and gentle awakening. We can begin crossing the abyss.

Yoga is many different things to many different people and it will continue to evolve with time. I am still learning and I am sure I will continue to make mistakes as I navigate this ancient spiritual practice and discover more about its rich history and sacred traditions.

As more and more of us begin on this journey, may we restore yoga to its original wholeness, may we allow it to evolve while honouring its essence, may we embrace this healing and transformative practice as a way to know ourselves better—our fears, our hopes, our dreams, our privileges, our prejudices and our power. May we practise yoga as a way to move ever closer to peace, harmony and love.

The Seven Paths of Yoga

PEOPLE OFTEN IMAGINE YOGA to be about stretching and bending and creating a body that is stronger and more flexible with better balance. And, for most people, the body is the way in, the gateway to a deeper practice that encompasses all aspects of our lives: our body, our family, our communities, our work, our art, our politics and our planet.

But, there are many paths up the mountain. As well as the physical poses, there are numerous ways for us to practise yoga off the mat and to integrate the wisdom and compassion we cultivate during our physical practice into our daily lives. By following one or more of these paths, we begin a journey that allows us to get to know who we are, why we are here and what is sacred. According to wisdom contained in the *Vedas* (sacred Indian texts from which the practice of yoga has evolved), not knowing who we are is one of the reasons we suffer, along with attachment and addiction, trying to avoid pain, identifying with our ego and being afraid of death. The paths of yoga are routes out of suffering – practices that awaken love, wisdom and compassion within us, and, over time, help us become more aware, more accepting, less anxious and less afraid.

Many people focus purely on modern postural yoga when they begin to practise, specifically the poses, while some feel drawn towards exploring other paths too. Allow your intuition to guide you. Trying to capture the vastness of these paths in a couple of pages would be impossible, so below is a simplified explanation of each of the main paths, based on my own understanding, practice and teaching. As always, take what you need and leave the rest behind.

1 Hatha

The path of *hatha yoga*, the yoga of physical effort, is what most people imagine yoga to be. This path uses the body as a vehicle for awareness and transformation. Through poses, and breathwork and lifestyle practices including eating a wholesome diet, hatha yoga uses the body as a training ground to build strength, both inner and outer, and to develop discipline, wisdom and compassion. Sometimes, in the middle of a challenging pose, you will find your mind trying to convince you to give up. Thoughts, like 'This is hard', 'My legs hurt', and 'I can't do this', will race through your mind. As your physical practice strengthens and you journey deeper down this path, you will discover that you can stay in the pose even though it is hard, that you can be with discomfort, and that you don't have to listen to the voice in your head that says you can't do things because you aren't strong enough or smart enough or good enough. Because you are and you can.

2 Jnana

Jnana yoga, the path of wisdom, is becoming increasingly popular as more people become interested in personal and spiritual growth. It involves what psychology calls introspection, religion refers to as contemplation and philosophy terms self-study, self-reflection or self-enquiry. Much of *jnana yoga* is about reconnecting with who we are beneath the masks we wear: rediscovering our true Self. This often begins with the sacred question, 'Who am I?', which we can usually answer only by asking ourselves, 'Who am I not?'. My body, my thoughts, my career, my achievements, my possessions and my past are just a few of the things I have discovered that I am not by exploring *jnana yoga*. This is a path of unlearning rather than learning, a shedding of layer after layer of patterns and conditioning so we can know ourselves, our values and our gifts more deeply and, as a result, be able to offer these gifts to the world.

3 Raja

As scientific research into the benefits of meditation grows, the path of *raja yoga*, the royal path, has become more accessible. *Raja yoga* is a journey inwards using meditation to quieten the mind from the endless stream of thoughts and cravings so that we can discover who we are beneath them. By walking this path, by returning to our meditation cushion again and again, we can train our minds to find freedom from harmful habits and reactive patterns so that we can make conscious, mindful choices about our lives. By creating a sacred space where we can look at ourselves and the world deeply, *raja yoga* offers us a path where self-awareness can bloom.

4 Bhakti

Bhakti yoga is the path of devotion, the yoga of love. This involves the cultivation of unconditional spiritual love, often devoted to a god or goddess such as Ganesha (remover of obstacles), Vishnu (protector of the Universe) or Lakshmi (goddess of good fortune). But, 'god' can take whatever form you like and, for many people, practising *bhakti yoga* simply means having respect for all of life and treating everyone with compassion and love. For me, the path of devotion is about looking for the sacred in the ordinary and making everything I do an act of love. This path is about living a heart-centred life and using every experience as an opportunity to love – ourselves, each other and the world.

5 Karma

Karma yoga, the yoga of action, encourages selfless service as a path to relieving suffering – our own and others'. This often begins with an inner pull, a calling to do something of value with our lives so that others can find more peace and joy in their own. But this quiet calling to be of service often gets silenced because our rational mind convinces us that our tiny, humble acts of kindness cannot possibly make a difference. But they do. *Karma yoga* doesn't have to be grand, public acts of self-sacrifice. It's the simple, everyday acts of compassion, like washing the dishes and picking up litter, that become a way of doing our bit for the world. Practising *karma yoga* taught me that I don't have to save the whole planet, I can just take care of the tiny plot of land outside my back door. *Karma yoga* reminds us that no act of kindness is too small.

6 Tantra

A more controversial path is *tantra yoga*, the yoga of ritual. Tantra is often misinterpreted as a way to spice up your sex life, but it is actually about freedom, connection, intimacy, creativity and pleasure. By practising tantric poses, rituals, meditations and mantras, we begin to balance the masculine and feminine energies within us, and, by harnessing these energies, we can move through the world with more vitality, bliss and aliveness.

7 Mantra

A final path, *mantra yoga*, the yoga of prayer and chanting, is often practised in combination with other paths. Repeating a mantra or sound can help to disrupt negative thought patterns and focus the mind so we can be more present and move deeper into our practice. Much like music can calm or energise us, *mantra yoga* uses the vibrations of sounds to move energy throughout the body. Concepts such as 'energy' and 'vibrations' can feel very airy-fairy when you first begin your yoga journey, but often, as you practise these chants and mantras, you will be able to feel the vibrations for yourself and it will start to make more sense. The most common mantra used in modern yoga is the sacred sound, 'OM' or 'AUM', which is often chanted at the beginning or end of a class. To try it for yourself, position your mouth as you would to say the letter 'U' and then begin pronouncing 'AU...' with the shape of your mouth unchanged, finishing with '...M' as a deep humming (it sounds like 'ooooorrrrrrmmmmm'). As you chant it, you'll probably feel a subtle vibration of each sound moving from your abdominal area to your chest and then to your throat. It is these vibrations that *mantra yoga* focuses on creating in order to connect to the vibrations of the Universe.

You'll notice that these paths are nothing grand, mystical or otherworldly. They are simply ways to live your daily life with more peace and harmony. You'll find there is a lot of crossover between the paths of yoga and the weekly mindful living practices we explore in Part Two of the book.

The Ten Pillars of Mindful Living

IT TAKES COURAGE to look at ourselves honestly and see how – by accident, carelessness or exhaustion – we may causing harm or distress to ourselves and others. The ten pillars of mindful living, traditionally known as the *yamas* and *niyamas*, reveal to us where we may be acting habitually – out of fear, greed or selfishness – and remind us to be more conscious in our day-to-day lives, to pay attention to the intentions behind our actions and to treat everything and everyone with care and compassion. Including ourselves. *Especially* ourselves.

These pillars are not about good and bad or right and wrong but about living in a way that brings peace to ourselves and those around us and returns us to our natural state of health and wholeness.

We can also apply each of the pillars to our physical practice on the mat and, by doing so, we will experience more energy, discipline and body acceptance, and fewer injuries, less fatigue and less self-criticism.

The first five pillars are ethical restraints, simple things we want to avoid doing – lying, stealing, clinging, overindulging and causing harm – so that we can free ourselves (and others) from unnecessary unhappiness.

Compassion

Non-harm or non-violence, traditionally known as *ahimsa,* is the first of the ten pillars. And the best place to practise non-harm is with ourselves. If you struggle with self-care or have a particularly harsh inner critic, to treat yourself with compassion and gentleness can feel strange and self-indulgent. But, if we are to bring more kindness, compassion and love to the world, we must begin with ourselves. As our yoga journey deepens, we naturally become more aware of our inherent worthiness – who we are beneath our egos, masks and conditioning – and, by recognising that this inherent worthiness exists in other beings too, we no longer wish to bring harm to them either.

If we are to bring more kindness, compassion and love to the world, we must begin with ourselves.

2 Honesty

The second pillar of mindful living is non-lying or truthfulness (*satya* in Sanskrit). This means being honest with others and also with ourselves. The mind is brilliant at twisting reality to make it fit the stories we tell ourselves and this can lead us to seeing things as we wish them to be instead of truthfully as they are. *Satya* is about looking deeply at our fears and beliefs and asking ourselves some brave questions: what am I lying to myself about? What masks am I wearing? What harsh truths do I need to face? As we become more honest about how we feel, what we need and who we are, we reconnect with our true Self. And, from this place, we can realign our thoughts, speech and actions with our truth. Inwardly, we can learn to love the parts of ourselves that have not known love. And outwardly, we no longer feel the need to lie or speak half-truths. We learn to be open, truthful and compassionate and, in doing so, we give others the space to be open and honest with us too.

3 Abundance

The third pillar, non-stealing – or *asteya* – is much subtler than simply not taking things that aren't ours. The urge to steal or misuse what doesn't belong to us – possessions, ideas, energy, partners, time – comes from an inner void, a feeling of emptiness. When we don't feel we have enough – or we don't feel we *are* enough – we tend to misuse external things in an attempt to make us feel whole. Practising *asteya* involves remembering that everything we have is a gift and everything we need is within us. By recognising our wholeness, there is no longer an inner emptiness that we compulsively try to fill with other people's energy, attention or approval. Instead, because we feel whole, we naturally feel a desire to give – money, food, time – knowing that wealth is not how much we can get, but how much we can give.

4 Balance

Non-excess (*brahmacharya*), is the fourth pillar of mindful wisdom. This means practising moderation, neither overindulging nor depriving yourself but taking the middle path. Overdoing anything – eating chocolate, drinking coffee, running marathons, scrolling through social media – throws us off-balance. And self-deprivation – of food, sleep, exercise, nature, rest – can drain our energy and be just as damaging. *Brahmacharya* is about finding balance in a world of extremes; having a couple of your favourite chocolate-chip cookies without eating the whole box; watching an episode of your favourite Netflix show without binge watching the entire series; treating yourself to that cosy jumper without updating your entire winter wardrobe. By practising balance instead of overindulging on superficial, fleeting sensory pleasures, we open up space within us to feel a deep, boundless inner joy.

5 Non-attachment

Non-possessiveness or non-attachment, traditionally called *aparigraha,* is the fifth pillar of mindful living and final *yama*. Practising *aparigraha* helps us cultivate a healthier relationship with whatever we call 'mine' – 'my job', 'my husband', 'my money', 'my body', 'my friend' – so we can fully enjoy what we have without basing our worth on it or being afraid of losing it. Being attached – to people, possessions and beliefs – takes up space in our home, our head and our heart. In this way *aparigraha* is a practice in letting go. It doesn't mean that we can't own nice things or have grand goals, it just means our happiness is not attached to owning those things or achieving those goals. Every experience is better when there is no addictive attachment or when we're not grasping for more. Non-attachment allows us to love more deeply, live more fully, and, when the time comes, to gently and gracefully let go.

The second five pillars of mindful living are personal practices that focus on our relationship with ourselves – purity, contentment, self-discipline, self-study and self-surrender – so we can become stronger, happier and more loving.

6 Purity

Saucha – purity – is a practice of removing impurities from our body, mind, spirit and environment. As well as eating wholesome foods, looking after our personal hygiene and keeping our home clean and tidy, practising *saucha* is about being pure in our thoughts, words and actions; cleansing ourselves of harmful habits and recognising what does and does not serve us so that everything we do cultivates health and happiness. This means bringing awareness to when we are acting from a place of anger or obligation instead of a genuine desire to help, when we are being judgemental, and when our belief system and conditioning is getting in the way of us being the truest, purest versions of ourselves.

7 Contentment

The seventh pillar is contentment; unconditional acceptance; *santosha*. Society wants us to be unhappy with what we have so that we want more, work more, achieve more, buy more and consume more. *Santosha* is the opposite. It is the practice of acceptance – of who we are, what we have and whatever we are experiencing in this moment. This doesn't mean giving up on goals or no longer working towards change. We can both accept our body as it is right now *and* invest time and energy into its transformation. We can be content with where we are in our career *and* work hard towards getting a promotion. We can accept that we have only 10 minutes a day to meditate right now *and* long for more time to dedicate to silence in the future. As we find contentment with who we are and what we have, any aspirations for the future simply enhance our joy in the present.

8 Self-discipline

Traditionally known as *tapas*, self-discipline is the eighth pillar of mindful living. *Tapas* literally means to 'heat', 'shine', 'fire', 'change', 'transform'. And it is only with this fiery determination that we can bring about deep and meaningful change and transform our pain into something beautiful. It takes discipline and dedication in order to bring about change – whether it be stopping smoking, losing weight, writing a book, choosing a different career path, or releasing your harsh inner critic and cultivating inner kindness and self-compassion instead – and we can practise *tapas* in any area of our life that requires effort. Whenever we get on our yoga mat when it would be easier to sit in front of the television, we are practising *tapas*. Whenever we do the washing-up when we are tempted to leave it in the sink until the next day, we are practising *tapas*. Whenever we speak to ourselves with kindness when we would usually be cruel, we are practising *tapas*. Whenever we are acting with enthusiasm, determination and focus, we are practising *tapas*. And it is with this discipline – this fire of transformation – that we will free ourselves from stress and suffering and experience the flaming fullness of our lives.

Our yoga practice becomes one continuous process of remembering, of coming home to ourselves again and again, of relearning our worthiness and realising we are not in this world alone.

10 Self-surrender

The most challenging of all the ten pillars of mindful living is self-surrender, traditionally called *ishvara pranidhana. W*e have been taught to believe that struggle, control and micromanaging every part of our life – from how many calories we eat to how other people behave – is necessary for success and happiness. But, by attempting to control everything, we enjoy nothing. Attempting to control our diet, our body, our emotions and our relationships gives us a false sense of power. We may feel productive at the time, but afterwards we are left feeling drained and disappointed. *Ishvara pranidhana* is the practice of 'trustful surrender to god'. Trusting life instead of fighting it, surrendering our selfish desires for a greater purpose, and cultivating a deep and trusting relationship with our intuition, each other and the Universe. 'God' is a delicate word and many people feel uncomfortable using it. In yoga, god isn't a religious concept – it definitely isn't an old bearded man in the sky guarding the gates to heaven as I was brought up to believe – but simply the sense of being a part of something bigger. You can call this *something* whatever you like – god, the Universe, Big Love, Mother Nature, the Tao, creative power, connectedness, oneness, collective consciousness or simply our shared humanity. It is this *something* we surrender to. And surrender isn't some airy-fairy concept, but a personal practice that could look like anything from deleting the calorie-counting app on your phone to trusting your employees and delegating tasks instead of trying to do them all yourself. Practising *ishvara pranidhana* means we stop exhausting ourselves trying to swim upstream and let the natural flow of life carry us.

It can take a lifetime to understand these practices fully. And, as humans, we will repeatedly forget to practise them in our daily lives. As mindful as I try to be, I continue to forget many times each day. In this way, our yoga practice becomes one continuous process of remembering, of coming home to ourselves again and again, of relearning our worthiness and realising we are not in this world alone.

9 Self-study

The ninth pillar is self-study, or *svadhyaya* – which literally means, to 'recollect', to 'remember'. This is any practice – such as journalling, reading poetry and meditating – that helps you get to know who you really are: the true Self that glitters at the deepest core of your being. One of the most profound periods of my life was shortly after my Dad died and, every morning, I would sit on my sofa with a steaming mug of lemon and ginger tea and read a verse of the *Tao Te Ching*, an ancient spiritual text by Taoist philosopher Lao Tzu. I would contemplate each verse, journal about it, feel whatever sadness and fear came up and allow the words to serve as a gateway for self-reflection: who am I? What is my purpose? Where am I creating suffering and dissatisfaction in my life and how can I free myself from it? What am I willing to dedicate my life to? How can I share my gifts with the world? Those precious sunlit mornings, swimming through the icy waters of grief, were my own way of practising *svadhyaya.* Those gentle moments of self-reflection became a stepping stone to the peace and wholeness I live with now. By giving ourselves a soft space each day to slow down and breathe deeply and reflect on who we are and who we want to be, we can discover a whole new way of being in the world – one where the ever-present self-criticism and subtle self-hate softens and self-compassion and self-acceptance begins to grow.

The Five Branches of Health

IN THE MODERN WORLD, our health is often reduced to a numbers game – weight, BMI, step count, calories. We have watches that track our heart rate, phones that measure how far we walk and scales that calculate our body-fat percentage. And yet many of us have forgotten what it is like to *feel* healthy. To be in a direct, caring, sensuous relationship with our body. To care for our mental health in a way that allows us to live with greater awareness and acceptance. To experience the deep, spiritual joy that comes with living a life of meaning and purpose.

So much conversation around health revolves around the quest for perfection – the perfect diet, the perfect exercise programme, the perfect body, the perfect supplement regime, the perfect morning routine. But, when we take a broader view, we see that health is the opposite of perfection. It is, instead, a journey towards wholeness. It is not about overcoming our appetite in the hope of sculpting the perfect body or suppressing our feelings in the hope we become the perfect partner, but about reconnecting with and paying attention to every part of ourselves – our cellulite, our scars, our attachments, our intuitions, our ego desires, our dreams and our fears.

Being healthy involves paying attention to the *whole* of life – mind, body, spirit, relationships and the Earth on which we live. And, unless we mindfully nurture each of these elements, we usually find ourselves neglecting at least one of them, leaving us feeling imbalanced, unhealthy or just a little empty. We might have been so focused on our physical health – on building a body that is fit, flexible and strong – that we haven't been caring for our mental health, leaving us drained, anxious and irritable with those we love. Or maybe we have been so focused on living as ecologically as possible – going vegan, avoiding all waste and campaigning against climate change – that we are suffering from nutritional deficiencies and have no time to share with our family.

Each branch of health is intimately intertwined with the other. And, only by caring for all of them can we feel healthy, happy and whole. At its core, this journey towards wholeness, this loving nurturing of our mind, body, spirit, relationships and Earth, is the practice of yoga.

The yoga journey in Part Two of the book includes practices to nourish all five branches of health, each described in more detail here.

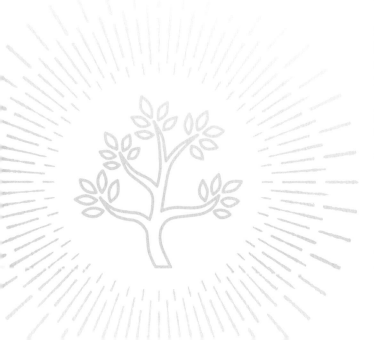

Health is the opposite of perfection. It is, instead, a journey towards wholeness.

Body

Many of us are called to yoga by a desire to improve our physical health; to become stronger or more flexible; to feel fitter and more energised with better balance and less fatigue. Research on the physical practice – the *asanas* – suggests that yoga can improve a variety of health measures including cardiovascular health, blood glucose and cortisol levels, oxidative stress, upper body, leg, and abdominal strength, and flexibility as well as improving sleep and reducing pain.

Hypnotised by diet culture, consciously or subconsciously, many of us are also called to yoga as a way to control our size and shape. Many of the messages in the wellness world encourage us to dominate the body. To master it. To control it. To treat it like a sculpture. A dumbbell. A machine. Yoga invites us to be in our body in a more compassionate way. To surrender our hard-earned power over body so that we can experience the power that lives within it.

The body as the first pillar of health is therefore not only about being physically healthy, but also having a healthy relationship with our physical self. One where we have the courage to embrace all of our body – its wisdom and its wounds, its strength and its scars, its wrinkles and its wobbly bits. But, in a society that profits from our self-hate, it takes courage to stop the war inside. To make peace with our body instead of fighting it. To welcome the parts of ourselves that have not known love – the soft curves and sharp edges wrapped in shame and unworthiness. Our corporate, consumerist culture encourages us to exploit and misuse our bodies – to diet to make them look the way the models in the magazines look, to push them beyond their limits in the gym for the sake of athleticism, to fill them with caffeine so we can put in 16 hours at the office, to eat foods that don't agree with us because we don't make time to cook, to refuse to rest even though we are exhausted.

Many of us spend so much time living in our head – thinking, planning, analysing, ruminating and worrying – that we have become totally alienated from our body. We may spend a great deal of time thinking about our body – what we'd like to change, where it hurts – but very little time actually living in it.

Our task is to come home to our body once more. To reclaim it. To reconnect with it, not as something to look at, but as something to live in. To relearn its wisdom, its beauty, its loveliness. Yoga is an invitation for us to let go of judgements about how our body should look and instead to experience it directly. Nakedly. To explore it with awareness. To surrender

> Our task is to come home to our body once more. To reclaim it. To reconnect with it, not as something to look at, but as something to live in.

to its mysteries. To live in it in a non-judgemental way. In yoga, our body becomes our guide. Our teacher. Our friend. As we practise, it begins to show us things – communicating not with words but with sensations, images, intuitions, feelings, tension, pain and somatic memories (sensory-based memories that are triggered by touch, taste, smell, sound and specific stretches and movements). When we listen to it, the body gives us a totally different way of knowing the world. Yoga is a pathway back into our bodies; to feeling and honouring the deep truth that lives within us; to becoming fully embodied; to becoming completely at one with who we are.

Like many young women and men, I spent much of my teenage years at war with my body. One of the gifts yoga has given me is showing me that my body is not an enemy that I need to fight or a beast that I need to tame, but a force filled with wisdom, that is loving, reliable and worthy of my deepest devotion. Yours is too.

2 Mind

If anxiety made a sound, the whole world would be humming. The breathless pace of modern life means that over 80 per cent of people admit to feeling stressed, overwhelmed and exhausted. And this is another reason why many of us are called to the yoga mat. We need an island of relief among the chaos of our lives where we can slow down, breathe deeply and listen inwardly. We need a sacred space to release, restore and remember who we are and what is important in our lives.

Our mental health is inseparable from our physical health. So much so that science has developed a branch of physiology called 'psychophysiology' to research the link between our immune, nervous and endocrine systems and our psychological and emotional well-being. On an even deeper level, Eastern wisdom embraces a single *bodymind* where physical and mental health not only influence each other but are indivisible from each other.

After decades of being a taboo topic, mental health is finally being spoken about more openly and researched more widely. Studies not only suggest that practising yoga reduces mental illness – including depression, anxiety and post-traumatic stress disorder – but that it also contributes to human flourishing: living an authentic life that brings inner joy and happiness through developing meaningful relationships, finding purpose, sharing our strengths and gifts, and being deeply connected with life as we journey through its peaks and valleys.

I think it's important to note that we can be struggling with our mental health and still be flourishing. Being able to embrace these apparent paradoxes of life is one of the greatest gifts of yoga. We can be going through depression *and* feel deep, inner joy. We can be in pain *and* feel at peace. We can feel broken *and* know at our core there is a place inside that is unbreakable. We can let in beauty even when we are suffering. We can walk through the world holding grief in one hand and gratitude in the other, allowing our hearts to be stretched wide by love and loss. Sorrow gives us roots. Joy gives us branches.

It often feels as though society promotes mental health as feeling happy all the time. It encourages us to 'get over' our grief, medicate our sadness and suppress our pain – often by distracting ourselves with social media, food, alcohol, television and online shopping. But mental health is about wholeness too: welcoming the *whole* spectrum of human emotions – grief, rage, love, pain, anger, frustration, joy, hope – and letting them pass through us. Yoga gives us a sacred space that might not be free from pain, sorrow and rage, but does provide the freedom to feel these vulnerable emotions without being overwhelmed by them; to be with the loss and the loneliness and to visit those dark places without fear of being trapped there. There is a lot you can learn in the darkness.

Mental health also involves thinking, learning, memory, attention and motivation. It means learning how to use our mind consciously instead of letting our automatic mind – our monkey mind full of cravings, addictions and aversions – use us. As we do this, we discover that we have the freedom to choose how to act. By following the eightfold path of yoga (*see* pp. 16–18) and exploring the many practices it gives us, we begin to train our mind so that we can focus for longer, think more clearly, and live consciously from a place of wisdom and compassion instead of reacting unconsciously, driven by our fears, habits or conditioning.

One thing has a more powerful influence on our mental health than anything else: mindfulness. Mindfulness is a conscious practice (for example, mindfulness meditation), a mental state of non-judgemental awareness grounded in the present moment, a therapeutic technique of acknowledging and accepting one's feelings, thoughts and physical sensations unconditionally, and also a way of being – a conscious, openhearted way of living with awareness, kindness, curiosity, patience and total acceptance of life as it unfolds from moment to moment. We will explore different elements of mindfulness as a practice and a way of living in Part Two.

3 Spirit

Spiritual health is broad and rich and deep and almost impossible to define. Ask ten people what spirituality is and you'll get ten different responses. To some, spirituality implies a connection to a higher power, a universal consciousness. To others, it's intertwined with religion. And to many people, a spiritual life is nothing otherworldly but living with a sense of purpose, belonging and wholeness. In practice, spirituality has very little to do with who or what you believe and is instead about how conscious you are and whether you are living in alignment with your values.

Our understanding of spirituality is personal to each of us and unfolds very slowly. The word itself, 'spirit', comes from the Latin *spiritus*, meaning 'breath'. In this way, the spirit is the breath of life – our lifeforce, our inner power, our creative passion, a miraculous loving force that exists beyond the boundaries of our ego. So, when we cleave off this part of ourselves, when we neglect our spiritual health for fear of being seen as 'hippie' or 'woo-woo', we are left with a void, an emptiness, a longing for wholeness.

Many of us live in spiritual poverty. Mother Teresa famously said that poverty in the West was not one of physical hunger, but a hunger for love, a hunger for god – not a religious, supernatural god necessarily, but an inner god, an inner peace, an inner freedom, an unconditional love that lives inside every single one of us: our spirit.

One of the reasons many of us overlook our spiritual health is because we don't really know what it is or how to nourish it. But, as the link between spirituality and physical and mental well-being has become impossible to ignore, science has begun to explore it. And while, at its essence, spirituality is an inner experience – an embodied knowledge – and therefore cannot be put into words, this more conceptual, psychological understanding allows each of us to care for our spiritual health in a way that doesn't feel so bewildering or overwhelming.

Modern spirituality is composed of three components: self-evolution, self-actualisation and transcendence. Self-evolution is a way of being where we are continually growing, deepening and becoming more conscious. Where we are awakening to our values and our purpose. Where we can let go of who we once were and open up to the never-ending journey of becoming. Self-actualisation is the process of becoming our true Self; of realising our potential – creatively, intellectually, socially; of sharing our gifts and using talents to do everything we can possibly do and be everything we can possibly be. Transcendence is the experience of wholeness, an acceptance and integration of all parts of ourselves – even the parts that are difficult to love. It is a way of being in which, underneath the everyday traumas and pains of life, we live with a deep, inner joy because we feel connected to and trust in something greater than ourselves. It is a way of living in which we treat ourselves and each other as sacred.

Part Two of the book will introduce several practices to nourish your spiritual health, each based around the spiritual determinants of health – the underlying aspects that cultivate the connection and wholeness we all long for. These include introspection, creativity, honesty, empathy, courage, philanthropy, humour, appreciation of beauty, questioning injustice, purpose, compassion, selfless action and having faith in a power greater than ourselves.

What humbles me again and again on my own spiritual journey is how very human it all is. Once upon a time I thought spirituality was something ethereal and otherworldly, but what I'm discovering is how spirituality is deeply rooted in this body, on this Earth, in day-to-day moments that look a lot like ordinary life. Ultimately, spiritual health is nurtured by connection and intimacy with all of life – our body, our purpose, our pain, our hopes, our fears, each other and the natural world. And therefore, anything that spreads love, connection, healing, forgiveness and acceptance is both the spiritual work we must do and a source of deep, meaningful spiritual joy.

4 Social

We are born with a longing to belong. To receive touch. To hear words that soothe and comfort us. To be part of a family, a village, a community. We come into the world expecting to be welcomed with intimacy, love and social connection. To know we are wanted and worthy. But, in our modern individualistic society, many of us go days with the barest of connections with each other and almost half of us report feeling lonely and isolated much of the time. And this loneliness epidemic comes with consequence in other areas of our health too. Research suggests that lack of social connection can be as damaging to our health as smoking and sedentary living.

Because we are born with an innate need for connection and belonging, when we feel deeply and intimately connected to others – when we feel understood, accepted and cared for – we thrive. We sleep better, feel more energised, have less physical pain and lower stress hormones, and we feel happier. Our close relationships provide us with a secure base from which to grow. They offer us a strong, supportive foundation that gives us the confidence to pursue and progress towards meaningful goals. Connecting with one another reminds us that we are not in this world alone. But, in a culture of increasing disconnection, where many of our interactions happen online, how can we connect more deeply, make our relationships more of a priority and create space in our busy lives for where love wants to live?

Most of us have some relationships in our lives that, with a little work, we can deepen. And, when we invest energy and emotion into these relationships, we usually find these people were missing us just as much as we were missing them. The ten pillars of mindful living (*see* pp. 22–5) can support us in developing deeper, richer, more meaningful connections in our lives. Whether it's a partner, friend, family member, gym buddy or colleague, by practising each of the *yamas* and *niyamas* in our relationships, we can connect in a more authentic way. For example, practising *ahimsa* – non-harm – in our relationships reminds us to treat one another with compassion, to become aware of the thoughts, words and behaviours that may be pushing a loved one away and then work towards transforming those behaviours. Practising *aparigraha* – non-attachment – in our intimate relationships allows us to love one another without an agenda, without expecting anything in return. Instead of using someone else to fill a void in our life, we focus on creating our own happiness and support our loved ones to do the same. And practising *santosha* – unconditional acceptance – allows us to accept others as they are rather than how we wish they would be. It doesn't mean that we don't encourage our partner to put the toilet seat down or ask our friend to be more punctual. Rather, it means that we are able to recognise that all humans have flaws and annoying habits and imperfections, and we can still love them – not in spite of their flaws, but because of them.

As our yoga journey deepens and we become more aware, more accepting, more compassionate, we often find our interpersonal relationships are transformed too. We discover that each moment of disconnection – every argument or misunderstanding – is an opportunity to move into a deeper love. As we practise, we begin to see that within us lives wisdom, strength and goodness. And, as we see our inherent goodness, we begin to see beyond others' flaws to the goodness and worthiness that lives within them too.

In a culture of increasing disconnection how can we connect more deeply, make our relationships more of a priority and create space in our busy lives for where love wants to live?

5 Earth

The World Health Organization defines three branches of health – mind, body and social – with suggestions to incorporate spiritual health too. But, over the last few years, I have realised the need to include a fifth branch: Earth. Because a gentle grief has been rippling through me these past few years, not a personal grief, but a shared grief – Earthgrief. It is a deep sorrow in my body for the suffering of the planet. I know I am not the only one who has been feeling it. You may feel it too. You can see it in the outpouring of anger at the destruction of the rainforests, the marches to raise awareness of climate change and the global rebellion calling for governments to reduce greenhouse-gas emissions. As much as we try to ignore it, the suffering of the Earth ripples through our lives, showing up as depression, addiction and the deep sense that something is missing, something we cannot name. What we are doing to the body of the Earth is reflected in what many of us are doing to our own bodies – depleting, neglecting and abusing ourselves for the sake of productivity and progress. A new branch of psychology called ecopsychology recognises the way in which mental illness and psychological distress is bound up with ecological destruction.

Healthy people can only blossom on a healthy planet. Because we are not separate from the Earth. We are part of it. We come from it. We belong to it. 'Shin to bul ee' is an ancient Korean proverb meaning 'body and soil are one'. The truth is, many of us have forgotten this. We have lost our connection with the Earth. And it's easy to see why. We live in concrete-covered cities and spend our days in high rise office buildings staring into screens, living as far from the natural world as possible. And it's hard to love what you don't know – the trees you have never climbed, the oceans you have never swum in, the wild blackberries you have never tasted. We cannot possibly face the destruction of the Earth (or of ourselves) without also remembering the beauty of the world and all there is to love. Ecotherapy – a novel form of psychotherapy that includes wilderness therapy and green exercise – focuses on cultivating a reciprocal relationship with nature: we nurture it and it nurtures us.

In the same way it takes time to learn what foods nourish your body and what self-care practices

> Healthy people can only blossom on a healthy planet. Because we are not separate from the Earth. We are part of it. We come from it. We belong to it.

nurture your mind, it can take time to reconnect with the Earth. For me, it's about living as close to the wild as I can. Getting down in the dirt and growing my own vegetables, composting, wild swimming, dedicating one day a week when I don't use my car and another day when I don't buy anything. I stay sober on a Saturday night so I can watch the sunrise on a Sunday morning and spend my weekends hiking up hills and exploring woodlands so that never again will I forget that I belong to this Earth and it is my responsibility to protect it and care for it.

The health, happiness and deep sense of belonging that comes with reconnecting with the natural world is the gift of yoga in the broadest sense. By practising yoga, by journeying within ourselves to understand our own dysfunctional ways of being and reclaiming our power to protect, to create, to transform, we wake up to the gifts each of us has been given to offer to ourselves, each other and this aching, shimmering planet.

The Universe of the Body

WE HAVE ALL BEEN TOLD BY SOMEONE – family, friends, strangers, advertising, social media – that we are too fat, too thin, too curvy, too muscular, too lean, too big, too old, too much. These comments can break our hearts and make us believe that our body is not worthy of our love and devotion.

Research suggests that over a third of us feel anxious or depressed about our body and one in eight of us has experienced suicidal thoughts because of body worries. We feel this pain because we've been taught to believe the body is an object to be overcome instead of a universe to be explored; something that needs to be conquered, controlled and shaped into a socially acceptable form. Cultural messaging places the body firmly in the category of expendable. Science treats it as a machine. Advertising exploits it as a business. The Church warns that it is the body that enslaves us in sin. And so, we find ourselves feeling trapped in a kind of flesh prison – alienated from our bodies, our emotions and the world, unable to see anything beautiful in ourselves, robotically skimming the surface of our lives instead of fully, fiercely living them.

Yoga gives us a way to reclaim our body. To reconnect with it. To relearn its strength, its wisdom, its beauty. The yoga mat becomes a sacred space to care for ourselves unconditionally instead of thinking, 'I will love myself as long as I have a flat stomach.' Through our physical practice, we move from the brain – and all its thinking and planning and worrying – into the wild mystery of the body, the only place where we can directly experience the vastness of our emotions and the richness of our lives.

Many people turn to yoga to help heal their relationship with their body. And my destructive relationship with my body was one of the reasons I first stepped foot on a yoga mat all those years ago. I had always thought being healthy required *more* control, *more* obsession, *more* struggle; that I needed to fight

my body because it couldn't be trusted. But, through my practice, I slowly discovered the body is not a battleground but a pathway to freedom. I let go of the idea in my head about what my body should look like and how much I should weigh and, instead, let my body be shaped by the things I love: yoga, handstands, walks by the ocean, homegrown vegetables, buttery apple crumbles and freshly baked carrot cake. By coming in to a direct, caring relationship with my body on the mat, I glimpsed how much more joyful and peaceful life can be when you let go of control.

It can take time to relinquish our hard-earned control over our body. And it can feel extremely vulnerable to trust our body and trust that everything will be okay when we do. But, as we let go of control, we will discover our body has a wisdom all of its own. It is our greatest teacher – better than any 'guru' or 'expert' or diet book. It will tell us when it needs food, when it needs movement and when it needs rest. Our task is to listen to it. To trust its signals. To explore its depths. To feel every emotion and trust every intuition. To awaken while we live in it.

Yoga doesn't make all our body-image concerns go away overnight, but it does give us a different way to relate to them. Instead of being things we need to overcome, our insecurities become gateways to becoming fully human. Not flawless, unfeeling, constantly productive superhumans but fully feeling, fully alive, fully awake humans.

Yoga allows us to embrace the *whole* body – the aches and pains, the tight muscles and injuries, the softness of our belly, the wobble of our legs, the deep sadness in our heart, the grief that clings to the wall of our ribcage. And from this place of unconditional acceptance, something magical happens: we begin to take care of our body in ways we might not have done before. We feed it nutritious food that gives us the energy to live an active life, we go to that dance class we always wanted to try but felt we were too big for, we make time for yoga and stretching and strength training, not out of fear of gaining weight or getting sick, but out of a deep love and respect for the sacred vessel that is our home.

Much of the yoga journey in Part Two of this book is a journey to embodiment; a shift from thinking and planning and analysing our lives to sensually, intuitively, nakedly living them. This is about moving from ego-consciousness – and the self-consciousness and self-judgement that comes with it – to somatic awareness: a way of being in the world where we are able to fully live the life that is arriving in our body, moment to moment.

As we begin our yoga journey, we have to be willing to let our body show us the way.

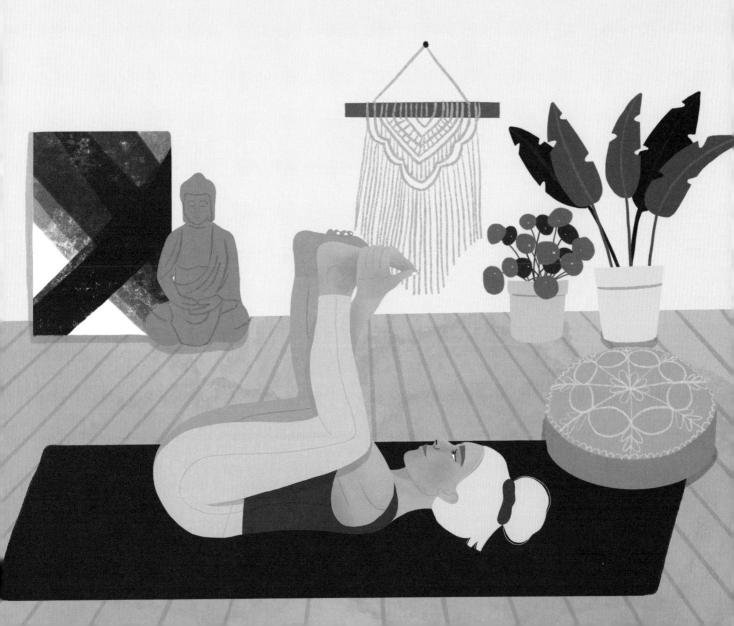

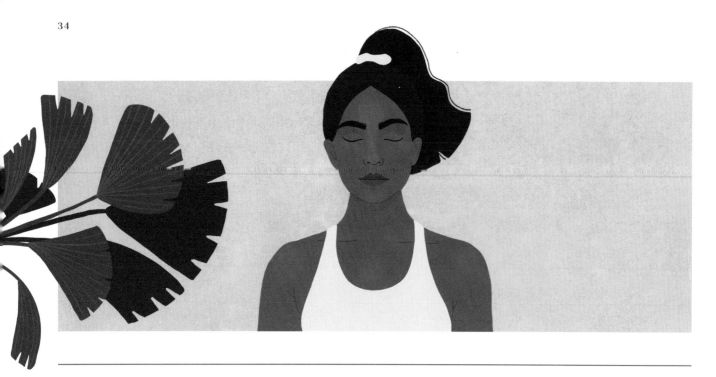

Breath is the Bridge

THE BREATH IS OUR BASIC CONNECTION TO LIFE. It is our anchor to the present moment, a doorway to our inner world, and a bridge connecting mind and body, conscious and unconscious, human and Earth. As we draw each breath inside our body, just for a moment, the world becomes us, and, as we exhale, a part of us becomes the world. But, as we increasingly find ourselves moving at a breathless pace, trying to keep up with the machines of our culture, we begin to lose our connection with the breath. We might find that we take short, shallow breaths and sometimes we might not be breathing at all – unintentionally holding our breath and clenching our jaw as a response to feeling stressed, anxious or overwhelmed.

When we lose our connection with the breath, we also lose our connection with our body, our emotions and life itself. We find ourselves trapped in the thinking, judging part of the brain – analysing the past and worrying about the future – instead of feeling the full force of life that flows through us and around us from moment to moment.

Reconnecting with the breath takes time. If we have spent years unconsciously restricting our breath because of stress or taking short, shallow breaths because of the cultural pressure to have a flat stomach, learning to breathe smoothly and evenly again is often quite difficult. Cultivating this connection with the breath is another gift of yoga. In fact, the starting point for our practice is always the breath. If we're not paying attention to our breath, we're just doing gymnastics on a mat. And, while there is nothing wrong with working towards headstands and handstands, ignoring the breath during our practice tends to leave us feeling completely wiped out – exhausted instead of energised, fragmented instead of whole.

Many people find it difficult to pay attention to their

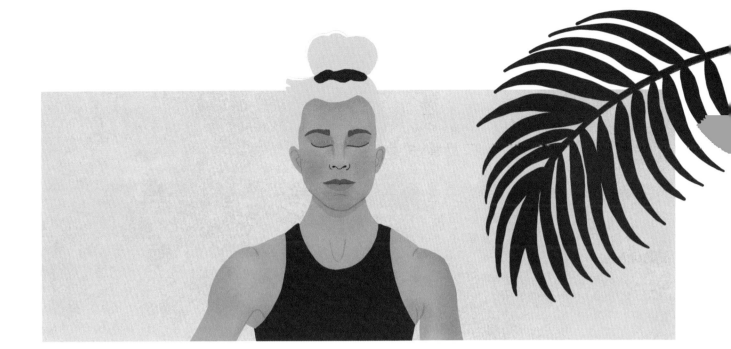

breath when they get on their mat because there is so much else to think about: which leg to bend, where to place your foot, how to move your arms without falling over. But, with patience and practise, we are able to maintain a smooth, steady breath throughout our practice, to keep our focus on our breath for longer, and when our mind does wander, we are able to catch ourselves more quickly and come back to the moment more easily. Over time, we discover that the repetitive nature of the breath becomes like a metronome – setting the pace for our practice and letting us know when to slow down, when to push forwards and when to rest. And, as our practice challenges us and we come up against tightness and tension, we are able to use the breath to soften into each pose and create space around difficult sensations and emotions instead of struggling against them.

With time, the breath becomes the background soundtrack for our practice and our lives. It is a universal, ever-present, beautifully simple tool that frees us from the chatter of our thinking mind so that we can experience life in a fully embodied, empowered way. There are several specialist yoga breathing techniques known as *pranayama* – some to calm and some to energise – which we will explore in greater detail throughout Part Two of the book, but to begin with, simply pay attention to your breath in everyday life.

Our breath is a reflection of how we are feeling – even before we are consciously aware of how we are feeling – so, whenever we notice the breath becoming sharp or shallow, or rapid or heavy, we can use it to pay attention to the anger, fear or frustration that is swirling below the surface of our lives so we can deal with it mindfully and compassionately. And, whenever our mind becomes scattered, we can use our breath to gently take hold of it and bring us back into the present moment. Because we cannot think and be aware of our breath at the same time, often, one full conscious breath is all it takes to interrupt the incessant steam of thinking and worrying that many of us live with.

The breath is a powerful tool. It allows us to explore whatever is unknown about ourselves. To escape our judging, thinking mind. To experience the aliveness flowing through our body. To ground us in the present moment. To guide us home to our true Self.

Create space around difficult sensations and emotions instead of struggling against them.

The Language of Yoga

ONE OF THE MOST CONFUSING THINGS about beginning a yoga practice can be wrapping your head around so many new words. What is a 'bind'? Where is my 'midline'? How do I create a 'neutral pelvis'? Below you'll find a list of terms that are used throughout Part Two of the book and that you may also hear when you go to a yoga class.

Commonly Used Terms

ALIGNMENT – the precise way to practise each pose to maximise its benefits and minimise risk of injury. There are universal guidelines around alignment but the more subtle elements will be personal to everybody.

ASHTANGA YOGA – an energetic style of breath-synchronised yoga that follows a set sequence of poses.

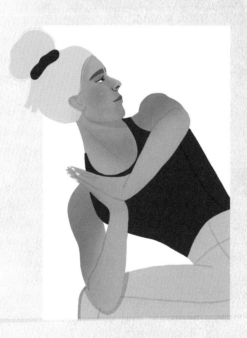

AUTONOMIC NERVOUS SYSTEM – part of the peripheral nervous systems that regulates bodily functions (such as heart rate and digestion). It's divided into two parts: the sympathetic nervous system (responsible for fight-or-flight response) and the parasympathetic nervous system (responsible for digestion and repair).

AYURVEDA – the 'science of life'. One of the world's oldest healing systems based on mind-body-spirit wellness. It aims to promote health – rather than fight disease – through diet, exercise, spiritual practices, herbal remedies, sleep, nature and relationships.

BANDHA – the 'lock' or co-contraction of muscles either side of a joint to create stability in each pose. There are four main *bandhas* in yoga explored on pages 50–1.

BIND – rotating the shoulders and linking the hands in a pose to create stability. For example, in Bound Side Angle Pose (*see* p. 105).

CENTERING — being fully present in your body by sensing the centre of peace and quietness within you.

CONTRACT – to activate or engage muscles. This can feel like tensing or squeezing the muscle to provide stability. The opposite of relaxing a muscle.

CORE – the central part of the body including the pelvic floor, abdominals, obliques, erector muscles and glutes.

DUMPING – the tendency to place excess pressure in to the lower back – especially in backbends – which can lead to back pain. This is usually caused by weak abdominals.

FLEX – used in relation to the feet to mean to draw back the toes – the opposite of pointing.

FLOAT—jumping and landing lightly in flows such as Sun Salutations instead of landing with a thud.

FLOW — a series of poses practised one after the other in a dance-like way, usually in sync with the breath.

FLOW STATE – an optimal state of consciousness where we feel and perform our best. A state of egolessness, timelessness and complete presence, where every thought and action flows effortlessly from one to the next.

FOLD – to lay the torso over the thighs.

GLUTES – the gluteal muscles. The three muscles that make up the buttocks – gluteus maximus, gluteus medius and gluteus minimus.

GROUNDING — being fully present in your body (often by sensing the ground beneath you) and/or rebalancing your electrical energy by connecting directly to the earth (for example, by walking barefoot).

IYENGAR YOGA – an alignment-based style of yoga that places emphasis on optimal position and precision in each pose.

JALANDHARA BANDHA – chin lock. A subtle tuck of the chin to bring the neck into alignment. *See* page 50–1 for more details.

LENGTHEN – a subtle extension of the spine practiced in poses on an inhalation in order to create space and stability in the spine.

MIDLINE – an imaginary line down the centre of the body from head to toe.

MULA BANDHA – root lock. A subtle engagement of the pelvic floor to stabilise the pelvis. *See* page 50 for more details.

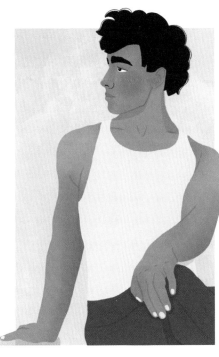

NERVOUS SYSTEM – the network of nerves that runs throughout the body (peripheral nervous system) as well as the spinal column and brain (central nervous system).

NEUTRAL PELVIS – the position of the pelvis when the top of the pelvis is in line at the back and front of the body and the left and right hips are on the same plane.

PRAYER POSITION — pressing palms together in front of the chest as a reminder to centre ourselves in our heart instead of our ego.

RELAX – taking all tension out of the muscle. The opposite of contracting the muscle.

RELEASE – a subtle deepening in the pose, practised on an exhalation.

ROLL OVER YOUR TOES — the transition from Upward Dog (where the top of your feet are on the mat) to Downward Dog (where the soles of your feet are on the mat).

SITTING BONES – the rounded bone in each buttock that we want to balance on in seated postures.

TAILBONE – the bone at the base of your spine also known as your coccyx.

THIRD EYE – the area at the centre of your forehead, often linked to intuition.

TRANSITION — poses or movements that help you move from one pose to the next.

UDDIYANA BANDHA – abdominal lock. A subtle engagement of the abdominal muscles which brings lightness and grace to movement. See page 50 for more details.

VISUALISATION — a meditative technique using imagery to harness the power of the subconscious mind.

WRAP YOUR TRICEPS UNDER – subtle external rotation of your upper arms to create stability throughout the shoulders.

YANG POSE – an active pose, usually held for 5–10 breaths, which builds strength, stability and endurance in the muscles, as well as increasing flexibility.

YIN POSE – a passive pose, held for 2 to 10 minutes, which targets the deeper connective tissues.

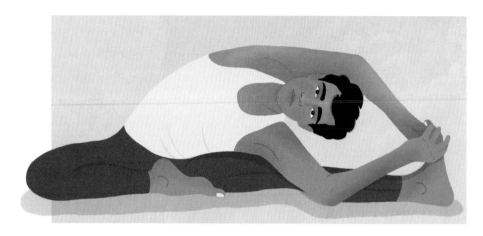

Sanskrit

As we begin our practice and learn how to move our body into poses, it can be helpful to learn some basic Sanskrit words. This is not at all a necessity but it will add depth and is a helpful reminder that yoga is more than athletic activity.

Sanskrit is the oldest language in India and many yoga teachers still use elements of it when they teach in order to reveal the deeper meaning of the teaching. Admittedly, when I first went to a yoga class and the teacher used the Sanskrit pose names instead of the English versions, I found it a little confusing and intimidating, so here you will find a collection of commonly used Sanskrit terms. The language itself is beautiful – almost poetic – and when you break the words down into their component parts, they make a lot of sense. Something I have found helpful is saying the Sanskrit name for the pose at the same time as practising it. The unity between sound and body helps you remember it and the meaning behind it.

General Sanskrit terms

You'll often find these words used in yoga classes and other yoga books. Some of them have no direct translation, so I have tried to provide as simple a definition as possible. You'll find some of the words sprinkled throughout this book. A little tip is to break them down into syllables and say them slowly a few times before saying the word all in one go.

AHIMSA – non-harm, non-violence (*yama*)

ANANDA – bliss, utter joy

APARIGRAHA – non-possessiveness (*yama*)

ASANA – 'seat', poses, the third limb of yoga

ASHTANGA – eight-limbed

ASTEYA – non-stealing (*yama*)

BANDHA – 'lock', used in poses to stabilise joints and direct energy

BHAKTI – love, devotion

BRAHMACHARYA – non-excess, neither indulgence nor deprivation (*yama*)

DHARANA – concentration, focus on single object (such as breath, mantra), sixth limb of yoga

DHYANA – meditation, effortless awareness of the present moment without judgement, seventh limb of yoga

DRISHTI – gaze point, where to look during a pose or meditation

ISHVARA PRANIDHANA – self-surrender, surrender to a higher power (*niyama*)

MANTRA – 'mind instrument', sacred sound

MUDRA – a gesture practised with the hands and fingers

NAMASTE – 'I bow to you', 'the light in me honours the light in you', a respectful greeting often said at the start and end of yoga classes. Pronounced 'Nah-mah-stay'.

NIYAMAS – inner observances, personal practices to cultivate a deeper, more compassionate relationship with the Self, the second limb of yoga

OM – the sound of the Universe (*see* page 21), also spelled 'AUM'

PRANA – lifeforce, the breath that rides the breath

PRANAYAMA – breathing practices, fourth limb of yoga

PRATYAHARA – withdrawal of the senses, reduction of external stimulation (such as, caffeine, social media) to help quieten the mind, fifth limb of yoga

SAMADHI – enlightenment, realisation, union, oneness, when meditator and object of meditation become one, living awake and consciously, eighth limb of yoga

SANTOSHA – complete acceptance, contentment (*niyama*)

SATYA – non-lying, truthfulness (*yama*)

SAUCHA – purity (*niyama*)

SUTRA – 'thread', aphorism, concise phrase expressing a universal truth

SVADHYAYA – self-study (*niyama*)

TAPAS – self-discipline (*niyama*)

YAMAS – ethical restraints, things to avoid doing in order to find freedom from suffering, first limb of yoga

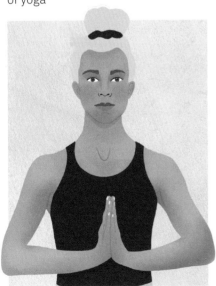

Sanskrit pose names

Understanding some simple Sanskrit words can help you access the more subtle aspects of poses. For example, the Sanskrit name for a Seated Forward Bend (*see* pp. 130–1) is *paschimottanasana*, which breaks down as *paschim* ('back of body') + *uttan* ('intense stretch') + *asana* ('pose'). By understanding this, we know that when we are in the pose, we want to feel an intense stretch to the back of the body. Again, don't worry too much about learning Sanskrit if you're just starting out – you'll find both the Sanskrit and English names alongside each pose in Part Two.

ANIMALS:

BAK – crane
BHUJA – cobra
GARUDA – king of birds, eagle
KAK – crow
MARJARI – cat
SVANA – dog
USTRA – camel

ANATOMY:

ANGA – limb
ANGHUSTA – big toe, thumb
BHUJA – shoulder
HASTA – hand
JANA – knee
PADA – foot, leg
PARSVA – side of body
PASCHIMA – back of body
PURVA – front of body
SIRSA – head

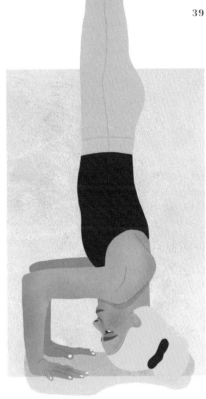

OBJECTS:

DANDA – staff, stick
DHANUR – bow
HALA – plough
NAVA – boat
PADMA – lotus
SETU – bridge
VRKS – tree

CHARACTERISTICS:

ADHO – downward
ARDHA – half
BADDHA – bound
EKA – one
KONA – angle
PARIVRTTA – revolved, twisted
PRASARITA – spread wide
SALAMBA – supported
SAMAS – equal
SUPTA – reclining, sleeping
TRI – three
UTTAN – intense stretch
UTTHITA – extended

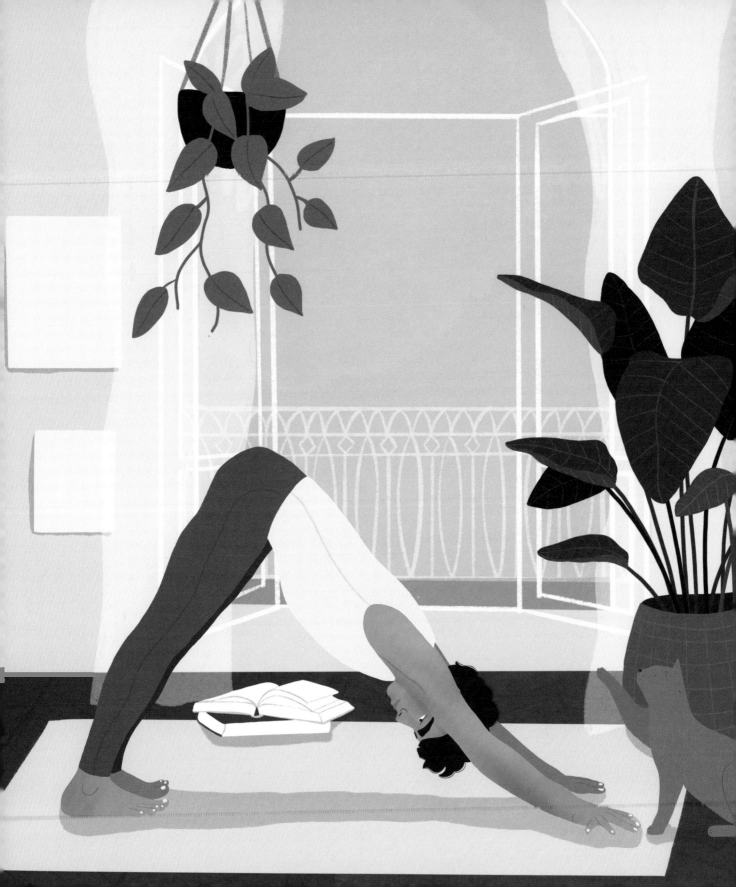

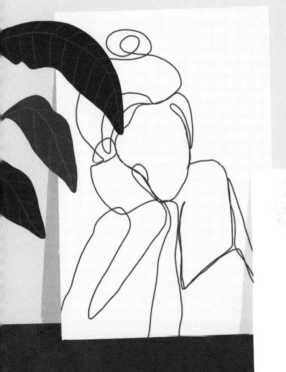

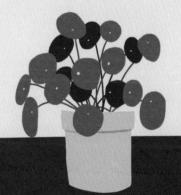

PART TWO

Practice

The Journey

THE UNFOLDING JOURNEY OF YOGA is just that. A journey we will be on for the rest of our lives. Do not hurry to reach the finish line, for there is none. Remember, we are not working towards some external goal or striving for a non-existent perfection that we hope to one day achieve. Rather, the practice of yoga is one of unfolding, unmasking, unlearning; taking off our armour and becoming more nakedly ourselves. The entire journey is one of becoming more and more who we are.

Sometimes the most difficult part of our journey is where to begin. So, what you'll find in this part of the book is a ten-week process that enables you to experience the transformative power of yoga for yourself. Each week will introduce you to a yoga sequence, meditation technique and mindful living practices based on the ten pillars of mindful living (*see* pp. 22–5) so that you can integrate whatever you learn during your time on the yoga mat in to your daily life. I offer this journey as a kind of map but, ultimately, we must create our own path so I encourage you to use it creatively, allowing your body and intuition to guide you.

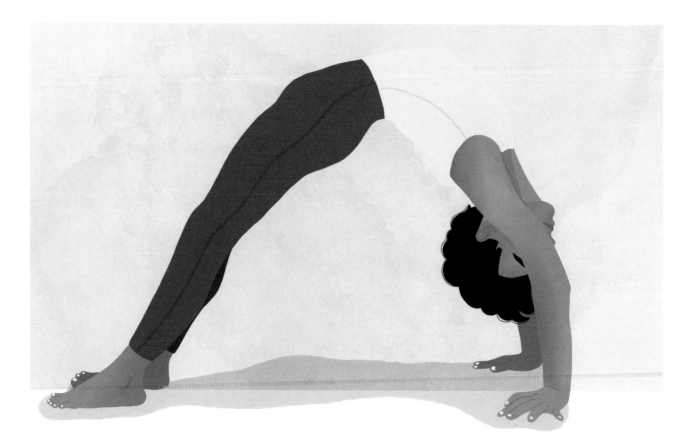

Yoga Sequences: *asanas*

There are two main ways we can develop our physical practice: in studios, under the guidance of a teacher, and on our own through self-practice. This book focuses on the latter, helping you to develop a strong, independent practice that complements any taught classes you go to alongside it. In my classes, I always encourage students to practise on their own too. The guidance of a teacher is often helpful – and sometimes essential, for example, if you are pregnant or practising with injuries – but self-practice is indispensable in developing self-awareness, self-discipline and self-reliance. Initially, you may feel unmotivated and distracted when you practise alone, but with consistent dedication, you will gain momentum and your commitment will strengthen quite naturally. Self-practice also has the benefit of being able to do it at home, at a time that suits you, with the option to adapt the poses depending on your energy levels, emotions and whatever you need in that moment.

The *asana* practice in the ten-week journey is made up of an opening sequence, a ladder flow – which we build by adding three to six new poses each week – and a closing sequence. The ten-week journey is designed so that you increase your time on the mat gradually – from 10 minutes to around 60 minutes over the ten weeks. By the end of the ten-week journey you will have memorised a routine that can serve as the foundation of your self-practice going forwards. The beauty of having a sequence we can practise from memory is that it not only means we can practise without constantly craning our neck to look at a screen or flipping backwards and forwards in a book to tell us what to do, but that it allows us to focus our awareness inwards and take our practice to a deeper, more meditative place. Practising from memory allows us to drop more deeply into our body – to practise in a fully embodied way – instead of from the thinking, planning part of our brain.

The opening sequence is made up of sun salutations – a traditional flow of poses used to warm up the body – and is how we will begin every practice. Traditionally, we practise sun salutations on their own until we can do them by heart and I would encourage you to do this with the opening sequence too. As you practise, you will discover the body has a memory of its own and most people only need to practise the opening sequence for three or four days before they know it by heart. There is more guidance on learning this sequence on page 10.

Once you can do the opening sequence by heart, add in the poses from week one of the journey. Once you have practised this sequence a couple of times and can remember it without needing the book, add in the poses from week two, then week three and so on until you reach week ten and have a full 60-minute self-practice. Although it's laid out in weeks, there is no rush. You may find that it takes longer than a week for your body to remember the poses – especially if you are only able to get on your mat once a week – so give yourself as long as you need before adding the next set of poses to your self-practice. This repetition is key to gaining trust in your body as well as building strength and endurance.

There may be days when you have time for only a short self-practice. On these days, I would suggest you do the opening sequence plus the poses for whatever week you are on (for example, if you are on week four, practise the opening sequence plus the poses for week four and miss out the poses for weeks one, two and three). Doing a shorter practice with full awareness is far more beneficial than doing a longer sequence with little awareness. And, if you are really short on time or fancy doing something a little different, there are some extra sequences in Part Three of the book.

Meditation Techniques

Each week of the ten-week journey will introduce you to a meditation technique. These range from mindfulness meditations to visualisations and body scans (a meditation practice that involves bringing your awareness to different bodily areas and physical sensations). If you are new to meditation, then simply begin with one to five minutes of meditation a day. You can do this after your *asana* practice, first thing in the morning, or whenever you find yourself with a quiet few minutes.

Most people assume that meditation is peaceful and calming but sometimes, when we begin meditating, we can be quite shocked at what we discover within us – judgement, hatred, anger, grief – and how little inner discipline, patience and compassion we have. When I began meditating, I was surprised at how much self-hate I discovered within myself. I had a problem with everything – too fat, too soft, too ugly, too pale, too wrinkly, too much, not enough. I discovered layers of anger and judgement that kept me at war with myself and the world. Underneath those layers were hundreds of layers of grief – for lost relationships and lost opportunities, for neglecting my body for so many years. But as I peeled back those layers, letting my meditation practice unmask me, I discovered a freedom: the freedom to feel, to love, to end the war inside, to forgive myself for all the times I forgot to treat my life as sacred. After spending years on the edge of burnout, trapped in an anxious and exhausting rush to nowhere, I discovered it wasn't my life that was busy, it was my mind. It wasn't the world that was exhausting me, it was my own thoughts.

In the same way our *asana* practice trains our body, meditation gives us a way to train the mind so that we can see ourselves, our lives and the world more clearly without looking at it through the lens of our fears, prejudices and conditioning. Meditation gives us a space to open up a conversation with our hearts, learn how to be with whatever arises in the present moment no matter how unwanted or uncomfortable, and, very often, to meet ourselves unmasked for the first time.

You will probably find that you prefer some styles of meditation to others. So, after the ten weeks be intuitive in choosing what techniques you use going forwards. Personally, after exploring lots of different styles of meditation over the years, I have discovered embodied meditation techniques such as Earth Breathing (*see* pp. 118–19) help ground me the most and then I weave in other techniques such as Loving Kindness Meditation (*see* p. 141) as and when I feel I need them. You may find a similar approach works for you.

Breathing Exercises: *pranayama*

I introduce five different breathing techniques throughout the ten-week journey – some fast, some slow, some calming, some invigorating. Much of the *asana* practice is what's known as 'vinyasa flow', which is the coupling of breath and movement; transitioning smoothly from one pose to the next in time with the breath. This means that you can practise some of the more subtle breathing techniques as you're doing the poses, while some are designed for you to practise on their own in a seated position. As with your meditation practice, you can either practise breathwork at the same time as you practise the poses or more spontaneously, in those quiet moments that open up now and then at random times throughout the day.

It's easy to underestimate the beauty of breathwork, because it often doesn't feel as productive or immediately beneficial as the poses. But I would encourage you to invest as much energy in to *pranayama* as you do on the mat because breathing properly has the power to transform your practice, your health and even your life.

Our hectic lives, often full of chronic stressors – money worries, work pressure, sleeping fewer than six hours a night – mean that many of us have an overactive sympathetic nervous system: we are stuck in fight-or-flight mode. Science has found that sympathetic nervous system predominance is associated with heart disease, high blood pressure, type 2 diabetes, obesity, depression, anxiety, fibromyalgia, irritable bowel syndrome and many other stress-related disorders. However, promising research also suggests that traditional breathing exercises have the power to rebalance the nervous system and activate the parasympathetic state – the optimal state for digesting,

Traditional breathing exercises have the power to rebalance the nervous system and activate the parasympathetic state – the optimal state for digesting, detoxifying, healing, regeneration and building immunity.

detoxifying, healing, regeneration and building immunity. As well as rebalancing the nervous system and having a positive effect on stress-related disorders, research is finding that *pranayama* can also improve several cognitive functions, such as memory and sensory-motor performance.

I find it helpful to do a little breathwork in the natural transitions of everyday life: a few minutes when I wake up in the morning, a couple of minutes at my desk before I begin work, or a few moments in my car as a kind of reset before I walk through the door. Yoga is meant to be integrated into our lives – not simply another thing added to our to-do list – so you might want to experiment with how you can create moments of stillness for breathwork in the natural transitions throughout your day too.

Mindful Living Practices: *yamas* and *niyamas*

Each week of the ten-week journey is based around a theme – such as compassion, honesty, balance and non-attachment – rooted in the ten pillars of mindful living (see pp. 22–25). This allows you to take the simple, meaningful wisdom of yoga and practise it in your daily life. These mindful-living practices are not complicated or grand. They don't involve huge amounts of time or energy or any big crusades to save the world. Instead they are tiny, intimate practices; the small acts of service that usually get squeezed to the margins of life in our busy, achievement-orientated world. Mindfulness is never practised in mighty or monumental ways, but in this moment, in the most caring and compassionate way. Many of these practices involve self-reflection so you might want to get a notebook you can use for journalling, exploring your creativity and noting down any realisations you have.

A Gentle Reminder

If all this feels like a lot to practise, then it's important to remember that yoga should enhance your life, not detract from it. If you can stick to a regular schedule, that's great. But if you can't – and many of us can't – that's okay too.

Be realistic about how much time you have to dedicate to your practice and allow the time you spend on your mat to evolve with the changes in your life.

You don't have to do everything every day – choose which parts of the weekly practice appeal to you the most and which ones you feel the most resistance to (we often resist what we need the most) and prioritise those. Equally, be honest with yourself about when you need to recommit to your practice and use a little more discipline. Some people create a ritual out of their self-practice – blocking it out in their diary and dedicating specific, sacred time each day or week to their yoga journey. This can range from 20 minutes twice a week to 90 minutes a day. If you know that you struggle with commitment, then you might like to make a contract with yourself, a self-practice promise, that will remind you why you are embarking on this journey. You can use the words below as a guide.

I, _____ ,
am beginning my yoga journey because:
_____ .

I commit to the ten-week journey in this book and promise to do the weekly readings and daily practices. I understand that some parts of this journey may challenge me physically and emotionally and I promise to listen to my body, give myself space for rest and reflection, and be gentle with myself at all times.

(signature)   (date)

As we find our own rhythm, we discover that a consistent practice is a kind of daily maintenance for body, mind and spirit, offering us a way to renew and restore, to release the traumas of everyday life and to remember what is truly important to us.

How to Begin

THE BEAUTY OF YOGA is that, other than a space about one metre square and an open heart, you don't really need anything at all. If you have room, you might like to create a calming practice space at home with candles and incense but if the only place you have to roll out your mat is at the end of your bed or in the kitchen next to the washing machine, that works just as well. Yoga is just as powerful practised in these small, humble places too.

How Often to Practise

When we begin a self-practice, little and often is usually the most effective. Partly because it's easier to fit into our often-hectic lives and also because it gives our body time to build the strength and endurance required for longer practices. If you're just starting out, I would recommend committing to three to four days a week of self-practice and then you can adjust this on a week-by-week basis depending on how your body is responding.

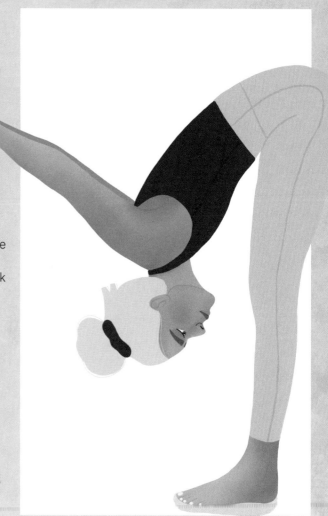

The opening (*see* p. 58) and closing sequence (*see* p. 75) take around 10 minutes, so you might do this four or five times a week for the first week to get you started (or even daily if you have time). Adding the series of poses in week one (*see* p. 83) will take you up to around 15 minutes of *asana* practice, which you might want to do four or five times a week to keep the momentum going and to help you remember the sequence. By week ten, the full practice will take around 60 minutes so you could do this three or four times a week or keep the full 60-minute practice to the weekends, with a couple of shorter practices sprinkled throughout the week.

The beauty of building our own self-practice is that we can fit it in around our lives and work with our own inner rhythms. Whether you do each element of the practice – poses, meditation, breathwork, mindful living practice – all together is totally up to you too. Some people like to start their time on the mat with a few minutes of breathwork and then finish off with five minutes of meditation and journalling or, if you don't have time, simply split up your practices throughout the day.

Equipment

While you can practise without one, a yoga mat with good grip will make your practice a whole lot easier and more enjoyable. There are hundreds of makes and designs to choose from to suit all kinds of budgets and you can usually pick one up in your local supermarket. If you can, opt for an eco-mat made from biodegradable rubber or natural cork so you can practise at the same time as protecting the planet. Some people also find using yoga props helpful – such as blocks, straps, eye masks and bolsters – but these are not essential. You can substitute with homemade versions such as using a belt or scarf instead of a strap and a thick book or firm cushion in place of a block. There is no shame in needing props, so please use as many as you need. Equally, it's easy to get attached to props and they can disrupt the flow of your practice so, if you choose to practise with them, use them mindfully – as stepping stones on your journey.

Clothing

There is no dress code for yoga, especially if you are practising at home. Simply wear something you feel comfortable in and that allows you to move freely. Wearing layers is a good idea as your temperature will rise fairly quickly during dynamic flows and then drop again during restorative poses. Overly baggy clothes can be distracting as excess material may fall over your face when you're upside down or fingers and toes might get caught in the fabric as you move. It's best to practise yoga with bare feet so that your toes can grip the mat but you might want to have some socks to hand for the final relaxation. And wearing a supportive sports bra is a good idea for women, especially in vinyasa-based practices.

Music

Traditionally, yoga is practised without music so that we can hear the rhythm of the breath. However, if you go to a studio class, you'll probably find they play music – sometimes gentle and quiet, and sometimes loud and booming – in order to set the mood of the practice.

I would recommend experimenting with both silent practices and music-based practices to see which you prefer. Some days you might find it easier to draw your awareness inwards without external music distracting you, while on other days you might find music motivating. There are some great mantra-based playlists online as well as songs based around sacred chants that many people like to practise to. Playing binaural beats – an emerging form of soundwave therapy – through headphones has also been shown to reduce anxiety and increase focus, so you might like to experiment, listening to these in your practice too.

Working with Illness and Injury

It's always best to check with your doctor before beginning any kind of physical practice or exercise routine. If you have injuries or are taking medication it's especially important to seek guidance from a healthcare professional so they can advise you how to adapt the practices to make them safe for you.

Pregnancy Yoga

This book isn't designed to be practised during pregnancy and, if you are pregnant, I would recommend practising with a qualified and experienced pre-natal yoga teacher – especially if you are new to yoga.

Common Sense

Ultimately, a safe, strong self-practice relies on common sense. Don't force your body into any positions it's not ready for. Don't push yourself through a dynamic, fast-paced practice when you're exhausted. Don't try and cram a 60-minute practice into 20 minutes. If you feel dizzy, sit down. If you feel pain during a pose, come out of it slowly. And, if you develop any injuries, let yourself rest. Remember, your body is your best teacher – listen to it, respect its limits and work with it gently, patiently, compassionately.

You and Your Mat: Practice Guidelines

Alignment and Aliveness

As we move through our practice on the mat, we want to find a balance between alignment and aliveness. This allows us to work with our body in an anatomically conscious way while also allowing for individual expression of each pose based on our unique body structure. Different styles of yoga prioritise different elements of the practice. At one extreme, Iyengar yoga emphasises precise alignment and encourages the use of props to achieve this, and at the other end of the spectrum, Ashtanga Vinaysa prioritises flow state – a meditative state of vibrant energy, creativity and deep connection – through the pairing of movement and breath.

The poses in the ten-week journey are sequenced in a biomechanically conscious way to allow for both full awareness of the experience of each pose and breath-synchronised flow. Some poses are held for five to ten breaths (30 seconds to one minute), while others are used as transitions to move through.

As I introduce each pose, I have included an image of the pose and general guidance on how to practise it to maximise its benefits and minimise risk of injury. I'd like to emphasise that these are *general* guidelines. If your pose doesn't look exactly the same as the one in the image, that's okay. There is no universally correct alignment and we should always adapt the pose to our body and not the other way around.

I would encourage you to release any judgement of how your pose looks and allow your body to find its natural alignment. As your body awareness grows, you'll notice where tension, weakness or resistance is causing misalignments. The body usually has a good reason for creating these misalignments so, rather than forcing

your body to look like the illustration in the book, allow it to realign naturally over time. We want to approach the poses with an attitude of ease and play rather than struggle and control. Your breath is a good guide to moments when you might be pushing too much: if it becomes fast and heavy, then relax into your natural alignment, no matter how the pose looks. Much of our time on the mat is about accepting our body how it is in this moment, not how we want it to be.

Loving Discipline

Yoga is about freedom. Freedom of movement. Freedom of energy. Freedom of choice. And one way to create this freedom is, paradoxically, through discipline. I like to think of the balanced, mindful self-discipline asked of us in our yoga practice as *loving discipline* – because discipline in our yoga practice should always come from a place of love, rather than deprivation, punishment or harshness.

Loving discipline encourages us to find a balance between dedication and intuition, intensity and consistency. It is loving discipline that motivates us to get on our mat on those cold, winter evenings when we are tempted to glue ourselves to the sofa and mindlessly watch television. It is loving discipline that reminds us it's okay that our first attempt at a headstand was not a success and encourages us to try again and again and again. It is loving discipline that encourages us to do the poses we find difficult as well as those we enjoy – to explore our weaknesses rather than avoid them – so that we can discover what our body's true potential is.

Sometimes when we begin a yoga practice, our passion can lead us to practice in an over-regimented, almost punitive way that leads to imbalance. If you find

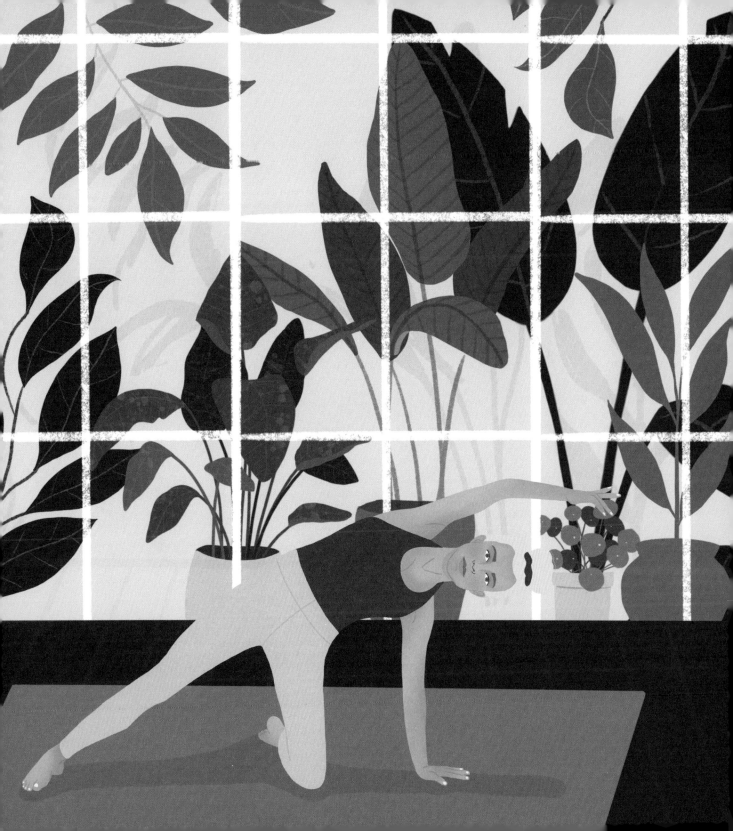

yourself slipping into this strict, ascetic way of practising, take a little break from your time on the mat and when you begin again, make sure that you are practising from a place of love and that freedom, joy and play take precedent.

Know Pain, Know Gain

Not so long ago, I walked into a gym and on the wall was a poster with the words, 'No pain, no gain. Shut up and train'. This aggressive approach to exercise is not uncommon. But, by disregarding pain and treating our body as a machine instead of the living, feeling, sacred thing it is, we are likely to cause imbalance and injury. When we ignore the messages our body is telling us – pain, fatigue, tension – for the sake of doing a certain pose or lifting a certain weight, we are operating from our ego instead of being fully embodied in our practice.

I have one rule when I teach: No pain. *Ahimsa* – non-harm – should always serve as a foundation for our practice. If you experience pain in a pose, especially if it's a sharp, shooting pain around a joint, then come out of the pose slowly. As our practice deepens, we'll develop awareness of various sensations – throbbing, tingling, aching, expanding, stretching, contracting – and different levels of discomfort. Our practice gives us an opportunity to explore these sensations gently and mindfully and, with time, we may come to learn that what we once thought was pain, may actually be a healthy discomfort that doesn't necessarily mean stop but is asking us to slow down, pull back and breathe deeply before we continue.

Staying present in our practice instead of striving towards ego-based goals is how we begin to differentiate between injury-inducing pain and the discomfort that we may experience as we gain strength and flexibility. It is this embodied awareness that will allow our practice to deepen, evolve and progress.

Bandhas

Our *asana* practice is challenging enough without applying lots of other techniques. But having a basic understanding of how to use the *bandhas* – the subtle engagement of certain muscles to create stability – can enhance it. If you are totally new to yoga, feel free to revisit the *bandhas* once you feel confident in the general alignment of each pose.

Although there are three main *bandhas* in yoga – at the pelvic floor, abdomen and throat – we can create a *bandha* around any joint in our body by co-contracting the muscles either side of it. For example, we can create a *bandha* around the elbow by contracting both the bicep and the triceps at the same time (explore this by trying to bend and straighten your arm at simultaneously). This gives extra support around the elbow joint, which is especially helpful if you are hypermobile (that is, your joints can extend or flex beyond the 'normal' range of movement).

The *Mula Bandha* – also known as our root lock – is the activation of our pelvic floor, which keeps the pelvis stable. This is a very subtle movement that happens naturally at the end of each exhalation and will develop as you practise. You can explore it by bringing your awareness to your perineum (the area between your anus and penis or vagina) and, as if it is an elevator, draw it up to the first floor, then second, then third. It's important to allow total relaxation of this area too, so practise descending the elevator back down to the second floor, then the first floor, then the ground floor, and then see if you can relax it even further, descending down into the basement.

Uddiyana Bandha – also known as our abdominal lock – translates as 'flying upwards' and subtly engaging it is what helps to give our movements grace and lightness. This is also activated at the end of an exhalation by drawing the area above the navel backwards towards the spine as if you are wearing a corset. This happens quite intuitively as you lengthen your spine and will develop naturally over the ten-week journey and beyond.

Jalandhara Bandha takes place around the neck and throat by contracting the throat slightly and pressing the chin firmly down towards the chest. We use this in most seated postures to bring the neck in alignment with the rest of the spine. *Jalandhara* translates as 'net in a stream', referring to its energetic qualities and the yogic theory that activating it prevents negative thoughts from flowing downstream and poisoning the body.

Again, don't worry too much about *bandhas* to begin with and avoid using force in applying them. Simply bring your awareness to your pelvic floor and your abdomen throughout your practice and notice what's going on: what sensations do you feel? Are the areas relaxed or active? Does your pelvis feel stable? If not, how can you create stability?

Little Tips

Following the sequences

In each sequence, each pose comes with an illustration, its English name, a recommended hold time (in number of breaths) and the page number on which you'll find detailed instructions of the pose. Each pose is also numbered sequentially, running across the page from left to right – practise the poses in this order. In the weekly sequences, the opening and closing sequences, along with each previous week's sequence, will be illustrated with its own symbol – if you need reminding of exactly what the poses are, simply refer back to the sequence for that week.

Rights and lefts

Traditionally in yoga we practise each pose on the right side before the left side and I would encourage you to do the same. All instructions are given for the right side so simply reverse them when you're working on the left side. Some of the illustrations have been drawn on the left side because the alignment of the pose is clearer from this angle, but still practise these on the right side first. Be aware that in the sequences, poses are sometimes linked together so that you will practise three or four poses on your right before repeating them on your left.

Most of us have subtle imbalances and one side often feels stronger or more open than the other. Be mindful of any differences you experience on each side.

Wandering eyes, wandering mind

Alongside detailed instructions of each pose, you will find a recommended place to direct your gaze to enhance your focus and stop your mind from wandering: your *drishti*. Focusing your awareness on a fixed point helps to quieten the mind and remove any self-judgement so that you can stay with your embodied experience and allow your inner awareness to unfold. Common places to focus your awareness on are upwards towards the third eye in the centre of your forehead, the tip of the nose, the fingertips and the toes – all depending on the pose.

If you go to yoga classes, it's quite common to find yourself looking around the room and comparing your practice to other people's, which can either feed our ego or crush our self-esteem. Using a *drishti* helps to direct our awareness inwards and reminds us that our practice is our own.

Every posture is a core posture

At its essence, yoga is about wholeness. This means that, while some poses may emphasise hamstring flexibility or shoulder strength, we need to bring our awareness to the *whole* body in each posture. Drawing our awareness inwards towards the core of our body as we practise will help to protect our lower back and will also create a stable base from which we can move deeper into poses. There are some poses – such as Plank Pose (*see* p. 68), and Chair Pose (*see* p. 73) – that focus specifically on building core strength, but in yoga, every posture is a core posture. To ensure you are engaging your core and not *dumping* into your lower back by overarching your spine, use the following cues: lengthen your tailbone towards the floor, lift your lower belly upwards and tilt the top front of your pelvis backwards. You can apply these cues almost universally to all poses – from balances to backbends – to ensure your glutes and abdominals are active and engaged (because we spend so much time

Focusing your awareness on a fixed point helps to quieten the mind and remove any self-judgement so that you can stay with your embodied experience and allow your inner awareness to unfold.

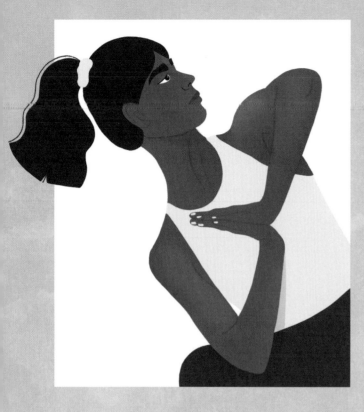

couple of hours before your practice if you're practising in the afternoon or evening and have a light snack like fruit if you're feeling hungry. If you practise in the morning and usually start your day with a coffee, see how it feels to practise without caffeine so you can allow the natural energy of your body to determine the pace and intensity of your practice. Likewise, notice how drinking alcohol affects your practice the following day and how your energy changes after a few days or weeks of being sober. There are more nutrition guidelines on page 54.

The final relaxation

In our chaotic lives, relaxation is highly undervalued. Many of us don't even know how to relax! Our muscles are constantly tight, our nervous system is in a permanent state of fight-or-flight and our mind whirs non-stop – thinking, planning, analysing. And, whenever we do stumble across a moment of peace, we often try and escape the intimacy of the moment by grabbing our phone or finding something to eat or planning what we're going to do tomorrow. Silence scares us. Stillness scares us. But it is only through these tender moments of surrender that we can fully know ourselves and fully love ourselves.

At the end of every practice, I encourage you to use the closing sequence (*see* p. 75). This includes *savasana* – or Corpse Pose (*see* p. 81). This is what the entire practice has been building towards and, although from the outside it looks like taking a nap, is often incredibly challenging. *Savasana* asks us to relax into our body, to surrender totally to the present moment without judgement, and to let ourselves be held by the ground beneath us. Letting go of control and settling into this silent stillness can feel incredibly vulnerable, but it becomes easier with practice. In the same way as you build strength with practice, you develop the capacity to relax with practice too. As tempting as it might be to skip, I would encourage you to do at least five minutes of *savasana* at the end of your session so that you can fully integrate everything you have discovered on the mat before rushing off into your daily life. *Savasana* is a beautiful reminder that yoga is not about improving ourselves or getting anywhere but simply about being fully and completely where we are.

sitting down, many people have 'lazy glutes', which often causes back and hip pain due to other muscles trying to do the work the glutes are meant to do).

Modifying poses

Alongside the full pose, you'll find instructions on variations of the pose that might work better for you – some will make it more gentle, while others will intensify it. Feel free to explore these at your own pace and move between them depending on how you feel when you step on the mat. If you're feeling exhausted, then take a gentler option. If you're feeling energised, challenge yourself with a stronger variation.

Eating and drinking

Use common sense when it comes to eating and drinking before your practice. Make sure you are hydrated when you step on the mat and be sure to drink plenty of water afterwards if you've done an dynamic practice. It's best not to practise on a full stomach so try to eat at least a

Self-care to Enhance Your Self-practice

SELF-CARE ISN'T ALWAYS SCENTED CANDLES and bubble baths. Sometimes it's a very unbeautiful thing. Sometimes it's going to bed on time, eating your vegetables and journalling about your struggles instead of running from them. Sometimes it's streamlining your life and giving up on some goals so you can dedicate to yourself fully to the things that really matter. These simple, unglamorous forms of self-care are things that will support and strengthen our self-practice. And, because yoga is not separate from life, any self-care that enhances our self-practice will naturally support our health, our relationships and our life as a whole too.

Sleep is a Superpower

Sleep is so important to our health and well-being that, if you have to choose between sleep and self-practice, I would recommend sleep every time. Adults need a minimum of seven hours sleep a night and some people need as much as nine or ten hours to feel and function their best. But, almost a quarter of adults get less than five hours' a night and one in two of us try to survive on six or seven hours on a regular basis. So many of us live in a state of chronic sleep deprivation that, according to research, is associated with an increased risk of heart attack, stroke, high blood pressure, type 2 diabetes, weight gain, cancer, Alzheimer's, and mental health issues, as well as reducing cognitive functions such as memory and focus. And experts warn that driving in a state of sleep deprivation is just as dangerous as driving under the influence of alcohol.

In a culture that promotes hustling and grinding as the path to success – and devalues the importance of rest and relaxation – getting enough sleep is hard. We are expected to work longer hours, commute further to get to work and to respond to emails around the clock. And, when we do get home (eventually!), we want to spend time with our family and read or watch a movie to decompress from the day so we end up sacrificing sleep instead.

Our corporate, consumerist culture means that we also tend to take a strange pride in how little sleep we can survive on, as if our productivity is more important than our well-being. Sleep is often stigmatised as weakness or laziness and we feel guilty if we accidentally oversleep, even if our body really needed that extra hour in bed. One of the biggest myths we need to unlearn is that sleeping is lazy. We know that sleep is a non-negotiable for babies, but we forget that it is a non-negotiable for ourselves too.

But, how can we prioritise sleep in our busy, over-scheduled lives? A bedtime alarm is a great way of reminding you when to start unwinding before bed. For example, if you know you need to be asleep for ten o'clock in order to get eight hours, then set a bedtime alarm for nine o'clock and focus the next 60 minutes on preparing for sleep: turn off electrical devices, have a bath, meditate, read. Going to bed and getting up at the same time every day is also really helpful for ensuring you sleep well, as is banning all gadgets from the bedroom, making sure your bedroom is dark and cool, and avoiding caffeine – such as that found in coffee, tea and chocolate – in the afternoon and cutting out alcohol before bed.

There is a deep power in reclaiming our right to sleep and rest. And once you feel how enlivening and invigorating it is to get enough sleep on a regular basis – and how much more focused and productive you can be as a result – getting eight hours sleep will naturally become a non-negotiable.

The Yoga of Eating

Nutrition is an emotionally charged subject. From vegan to carnivore and paleo to plant-based, most people have an opinion on what we should and shouldn't be eating. And many of us ping-pong from one diet to the next in the hope it will give us the body we have always dreamed of. All of this leaves us in a state of nutrition confusion. Are carbs good or bad? Is it healthy to eat meat? Is it ethical? Should we eat breakfast or fast until midday? Are smoothies good for us or are they full of sugar? Should we cut out bread? Is it ever okay to eat pizza? Or cookies? Or cake?

While having a basic understanding of nutrition is helpful – such as what foods contain protein, the benefits of eating fruit and vegetables, and which foods give us fibre – ultimately, your body knows best. As we become more embodied through our practice, we become more aware of the foods that energise us and those that leave us feeling bloated and sluggish. We can pay attention to when we are eating because we are physically hungry and when we are using food as a form of distraction or procrastination.

The fourth pillar of mindful living, *brahmacharya* – non-excess – reminds us to eat in a way that truly nourishes us. Neither overindulging in food for comfort nor depriving ourselves through harsh diets. *Aparigraha* – non-attachment – is also helpful to practise when creating a healthy relationship with food. Practising non-attachment in our diet allows us to relate to food with an attitude of openness and curiosity rather than obsession, suppression or compulsion. As our awareness deepens, we may realise that we have certain food habits that no longer serve us, such as using food as a reward, eating sweet things when we're stressed, and always going for the low-carb option because we're afraid carbs will make us fat, even though carb-free meals leave us feeling unsatisfied. This awareness allows us to let go

of attachments and develop a healthier, more mindful relationship with food.

As we let go of extreme diets and begin to trust our body, we usually stumble across the middle path: we feel our best eating plant-based wholefoods and earth-grown nutrients – greens, grains, legumes, vegetables, fruits, nuts and seeds – most of the time, but that triple-chocolate-chip brownie, or our favourite café bake, is exactly what we need every now and then too.

It's not uncommon that, at some point on our yoga journey, we forget that it's a journey towards wholeness and begin chasing perfection in all areas of life, including food. This can lead us to becoming trapped in orthorexia: an obsessive preoccupation with eating 'healthy' food. But any potential improvements in physical health will be outweighed by physical, psychological and emotional harm caused by neurotic obsession and high-stress levels. If you find yourself striving for perfection and following an overly restrictive diet, reread the pages on the ten pillars of mindful living (*see* pp. 22–25) and the five branches of health (*see* pp. 26–31) to remind yourself that *yoga is a journey to wholeness, not perfection.*

Intertwined with yoga is *Ayurveda,* a 5000-year-old healthcare practice that literally translates as 'science of life'. Ayurveda offers a beautiful, empowering way to eat because, instead of promoting the ultimate, perfect, balanced diet suitable for everyone, it encourages each of us to find a diet that balances us. For some of us that may mean eating lots of warm, grounding foods like porridge, soups and mashed potatoes, or we might feel better when we eat moist, unctuous foods like avocados, oil-roasted vegetables and buttery scrambled eggs. Much like the ten pillars of mindful living (*see* pp. 22–25), Ayurveda gives us simple guidelines so that we can tune in to our body and eat in a way that truly nourishes us: always sit down to eat, eat slowly and mindfully, eat in a relaxed atmosphere, avoid eating in front of the television or while driving, and try not to eat when you are feeling extremely emotional.

Remember, anything that leads to greater balance, wholeness and freedom is yoga. And as we find freedom from rules about how we 'should' eat and instead learn to eat intuitively – trusting our body to guide us – we discover how something as ordinary and everyday as eating is yoga too.

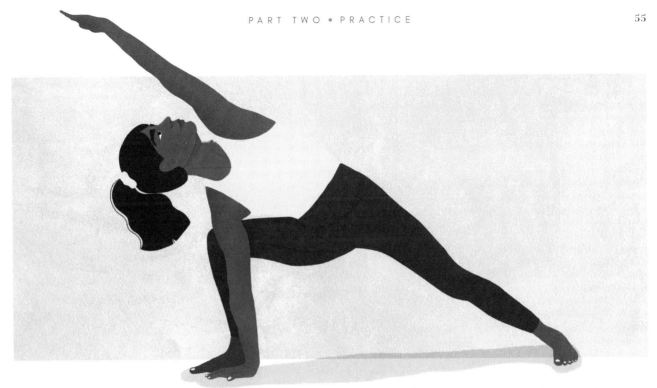

Moving for Joy

There are many types of exercise that complement yoga and give us the opportunity to both build and express the strength and power of our body. If you'd like to explore different types of exercise to accompany your yoga practice, my general guidance here is to find forms of movement that fill you with joy; that allow you to drop deeply into your body; that leave you feeling awake and alive. Some kinds of exercise can leave us feeling disconnected from our body. These are generally the ones that encourage us to disregard our body's need for food and rest in order to achieve an external goal – for example, weight-making sports such as boxing and physique-focused exercise such as bodybuilding. But, even these types of exercise, practised mindfully and with intent, can also be a path to wholeness. It is often our intention – the reason we do what we do – that matters most when it comes to exercising and working out. Are we spending an hour on the treadmill every morning in the hope of losing weight because we hate our belly? Or are we doing it from a place of deep love and respect for our body and a desire to look after it? Are we trying to lift heavier and heavier weights in an attempt to prove our worth? Or as an expression of and appreciation for our strength? Do we drag ourselves to bootcamp at 5.30 a.m. every morning because we feel guilty eating breakfast without working out first? Or because starting our day with a group workout in the fresh air leaves us feeling incredible? The intentions that underlie our actions plant seeds that grow into our beliefs and habits. Hate grows hate. Only love blooms into love.

Many people come to yoga in the hope of balancing out their body from years of intense exercise. Although it encourages a less forceful approach to movement, yoga will challenge you in different ways to the high-intensity workouts you might use. You might discover that your shoulders are tight and unstable from repeatedly rushing through workouts. Or you might find that you have lost mobility in your hips and lower back from years of long-distance running or cycling. Or you may notice everything is a bit wonky if you've always played a lot of single-arm sports like golf or tennis. After reaching a high level in our chosen sport, getting on our yoga mat and realising we still have a lot to work on can be a very humbling experience.

Whether you're keen to explore other types of movement to support your yoga practice, or have come to yoga in order to enhance your sporting passions, focus on using exercise as a tool to become more deeply connected to your body, your values and your life.

Writing from the Heart

What needs feeling? What needs healing? What needs grieving? How can we find balance in a world of extremes? How can we let go of the baggage that was never ours to carry? How can we take off our masks and become more of the person we'd like to be? These brave questions lie at the heart of reflective journalling – a practice that increases our self-awareness and helps us grow on both personal and professional levels. Like yoga, each question opens us to previously unknown dimensions of ourselves and our lives, to a deeper, fuller, richer way of being alive.

Research suggests that regular journalling not only improves our psychological well-being, but actually reduces cortisol – a stress hormone – when we're exposed to anxiety-inducing situations in daily life. Taking a few minutes every day to reflect on how we are feeling can help us to process and integrate our emotions – to move towards wholeness – and bring our awareness to areas in our lives that could do with a little work. Each week of the journey, you'll find a couple of reflective questions to journal on. These will help you explore and apply the mindful living theme for that week.

Reflective journalling gives us another path to freedom. To free the voice inside of us that yearns to tell the truth, that longs to tell our story. Writing in this way – without worrying about who is going to read it – is, in itself, a spiritual practice. Like yoga and meditation, it connects us to our deeper self. It is an act of listening to our intuition, our inner guidance, the tiny, tender voice inside; the only voice that is truly our own. Journalling is sensual, experiential, grounding. It gives us space to explore the depths of our lives and opens our eyes to another way of seeing ourselves, our experiences and the world.

Practising Together

Self-practice is wonderful. Empowering. Life-changing. But sometimes it's just as beautiful to practice with others. To breathe together, to move together, to awaken together. Every so often – once a week or once a month – I would encourage you to go to a yoga class and let yourself be taught. The simple act of releasing control for an hour and letting someone else tell you what to do allows you to experience the power of surrender. It might take trying a few different classes to find a teacher that you gel with and I would encourage you to explore various styles to see what approach feels most in line with the intention of your practice.

Yoga classes – and one-to-one sessions – are a really good way to get help with any poses you find difficult and get advice on any flows or movements you're struggling with. Sometimes a teacher will give you a cue or teach a pose in a slightly different way and something that didn't make sense before will suddenly make sense and you will be able to access the pose in a whole new way. Some teachers like to give manual adjustments in their classes – to help realign or deepen the pose – which are usually very subtle. They should always ask for consent to do this, but if you don't want any hands-on assists then make sure to let the teacher know.

Even in a yoga class, your body is your best teacher. If everyone else is flowing and you need to rest, then rest. If everyone else is attempting handstands and you're feeling dizzy, then relax in Child's Pose. If everyone else is doing big, deep backbends and your lower back is feeling sore, then take a gentler variation. Whether you're practising on your own or in a studio, leave your ego outside the room, and let your body and your intuition guide you.

> Taking a few minutes every day to reflect on how we are feeling can help us to process and integrate our emotions.

Let's begin...

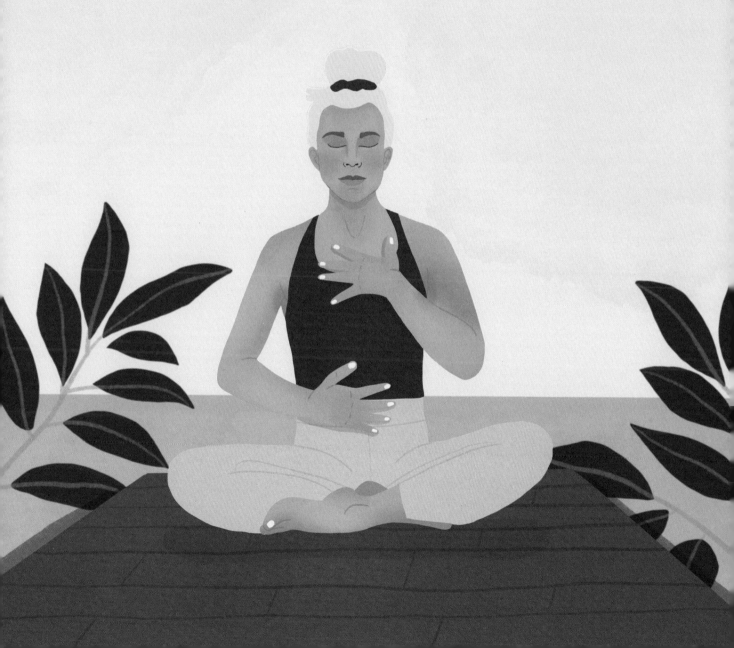

The Opening Sequence

The opening sequence consists of two variations of a traditional flow called a Sun Salutation. This is a series of poses that flow together to warm, open and strengthen the entire body. Traditionally, these are known as *Surya Namaskara* – meaning 'bow to the sun' – and were practised as a ritual of respect, thanking the sun for being such a powerful life source.

As you begin to learn the Sun Salutations, focus on moving in time with your breath – using Equal Breathing (*see* p. 62) or Victorious Breath (*see* p. 63) – and make each movement slow and mindful. Once you feel confident practising them, you might want to play around with the pace and experiment with how many rounds of each variation you do. I've suggested beginning with three rounds of Sun Salutation A and two rounds of Sun Salutation B, but feel free to do more or fewer depending on how energised you feel and how much time you have.

As well as using them as a warm-up, if you're short on time, Sun Salutations are perfect to use as mini-practices. Six to 12 rounds of each is surprisingly challenging! You can find detailed instructions on each pose in the Sun Salutation, as well as modifications, beginning on page 72.

Sun Salutation A

Begin at the front of your mat in Mountain Pose with your palms together in front of your chest in prayer position. As you breathe in, reach your arms overhead. Exhale and bow forwards, into a Standing Forward Bend. Inhale, lift your chest slightly and come up onto your fingertips into a Half Forward Bend. Exhale and step or float back in to Plank Pose, bending your arms and keeping your elbows hugged into your sides as you lower yourself down to Four-limbed Staff Pose (you can bring your knees to the floor here if you need to). As you inhale, push through your toes to shift your weight into your hands, straighten your arms and lift your chest to Upward Dog (or Cobra Pose if you have any lower back issues). Exhale, push into your hands, lift your hips and roll over your toes to Downward Dog (you can also use your knees here if you need to). Take five breaths in Downward Dog, making sure your hands are shoulder-width and your feet are hip-distance apart. Focus on lengthening your spine and creating as much space in the back of your body as you can. On your fifth exhalation, bend your knees and lift your gaze to look between your thumbs. Inhale, step or float your feet between your hands, keeping your spine lengthened in Half Forward Bend. Exhale, fold forwards to Standing Forward Bend. As you inhale, reach your arms overhead to Upward Salute. And, as you exhale, bring your arms back to Mountain Pose, either bringing your hands to prayer position or releasing them down by your side.

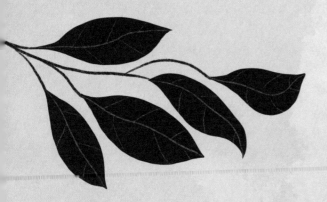

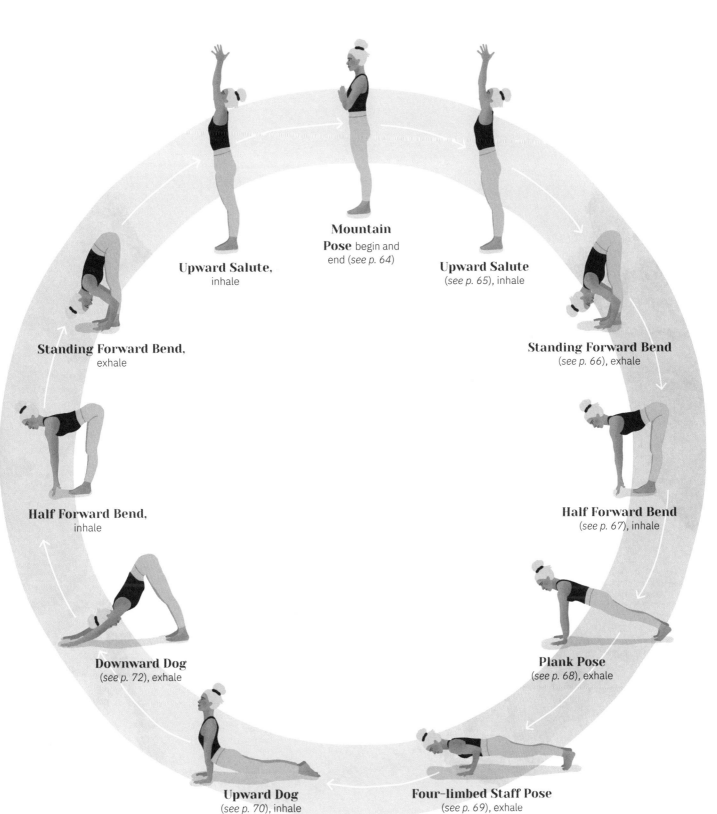

Mountain Pose begin and end (*see p. 64*)

Upward Salute, inhale

Upward Salute (*see p. 65*), inhale

Standing Forward Bend, exhale

Standing Forward Bend (*see p. 66*), exhale

Half Forward Bend, inhale

Half Forward Bend (*see p. 67*), inhale

Downward Dog (*see p. 72*), exhale

Plank Pose (*see p. 68*), exhale

Upward Dog (*see p. 70*), inhale

Four-limbed Staff Pose (*see p. 69*), exhale

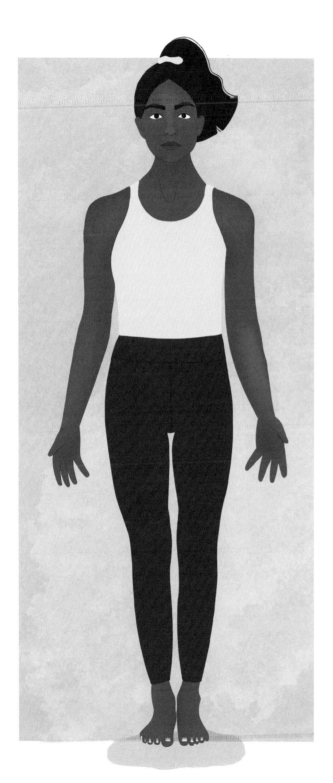

Sun Salutation B

Sun Salutation B is very similar to Sun Salutation A with the addition of Chair Pose and Warrior One, which help to create more heat in the body.

Begin at the front of your mat in Mountain Pose with your palms together in front of your chest in prayer position. As you breathe in, bend your knees, drop your hips and sweep your fingertips along the floor either side of you before reaching your arms overhead into Chair Pose. Exhale and bow forwards into a Standing Forward Bend. Inhale, lift your chest slightly to Half Forward Bend. Exhale and step or float back into Plank Pose, bending your arms and keeping your elbows hugged into your sides as you lower yourself down to Four-limbed Staff Pose (you can bring your knees to the floor here if you need to). As you inhale, push through your toes to shift your weight into your hands, straighten your arms and lift your chest to Upward Dog (or Cobra Pose if you have any lower back issues). Exhale, push into your hands, lift your hips and roll over your toes to Downward Dog (you can also use your knees here if you need to). Inhale, turn your left heel in slightly and step your right foot between your hands, lifting your chest and reaching your arms overhead to Warrior One. Exhale, bring your hands to the floor and step back to Plank Pose, lowering slowly to Four-limbed Staff Pose. Inhale and lift your chest to Upward Dog or Cobra Pose and as you exhale, lift your hips to Downward Dog, using your knees if you need to. Repeat with your left foot forwards and then take five conscious breaths in Downward Dog. On your fifth exhalation, bend your knees and lift your gaze to look between your thumbs. Inhale, step or float your feet between your hands, keeping your spine lengthened in Half Forward Bend. Exhale, fold forwards to Standing Forward Bend. As you inhale, bend your knees, drop your hips and sweep your arms above your head to Chair Pose. Exhale and release back to Mountain Pose.

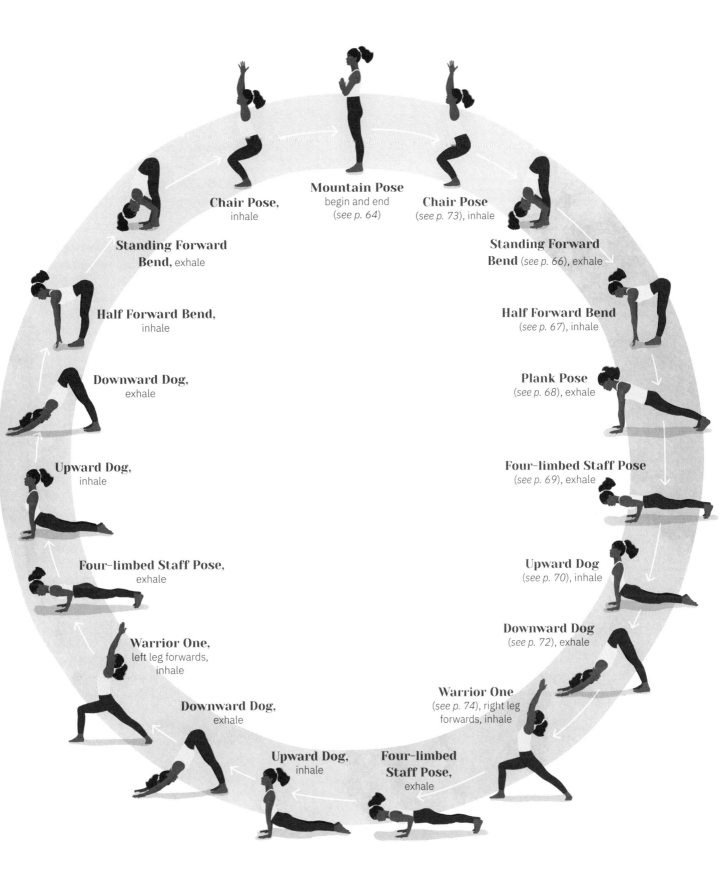

Mountain Pose
begin and end
(*see p. 64*)

Chair Pose,
inhale

Chair Pose
(*see p. 73*), inhale

**Standing Forward
Bend,** exhale

**Standing Forward
Bend** (*see p. 66*), exhale

Half Forward Bend,
inhale

Half Forward Bend
(*see p. 67*), inhale

Downward Dog,
exhale

Plank Pose
(*see p. 68*), exhale

Upward Dog,
inhale

Four-limbed Staff Pose
(*see p. 69*), exhale

Four-limbed Staff Pose,
exhale

Upward Dog
(*see p. 70*), inhale

Warrior One,
left leg forwards,
inhale

Downward Dog
(*see p. 72*), exhale

Downward Dog,
exhale

Warrior One
(*see p. 74*), right leg
forwards, inhale

Upward Dog,
inhale

**Four-limbed
Staff Pose,**
exhale

Equal Breathing

SAMA VRITTI

By making your inhalation and exhalation the same length, this breathing technique is both grounding and energising. You can practise it on its own as well as during your *asana* practice.

1 Begin breathing in and out through your nose, applying the same effort to each inhalation and each exhalation.

2 Establish a rhythm in which your inhalation and exhalation become the same length. For example, breathing in for a count of three and out for a count of three.

3 Allow a tiny pause at the end of the inhalation and end of the exhalation.

> **If you notice** your breath getting messy as you move through poses and flows, pause and re-establish Equal Breathing.
>
> PRACTICE TIP

Victorious Breath

UJJAYI PRANAYAMA

This breathing technique is both energising and relaxing. It involves gently constricting the back of the throat to create a soothing sound and generate heat in the body. It is often called Ocean Breath because the sound it makes is similar to that of rolling waves in the ocean.

1 Begin breathing in and out through your mouth. With each exhalation make a 'hhhaaaa' sound as if you're trying to steam up a mirror.

2 Close your mouth and continue trying to make the same sound. Notice the slight constriction at the back of your throat and the whisper-like sound and maintain this constriction as you inhale.

Use Victorious Breath throughout your *asana* practice. Listening to the soft ocean sound of your breath will help you stay present and focused.

PRACTICE TIP

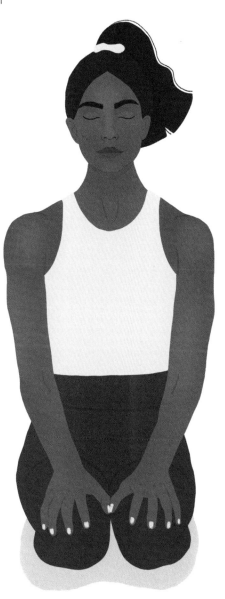

Mountain Pose

TADASANA

Mountain Pose teaches us to stand firmly on our own two feet; to ground ourselves; to reconnect with our body, our strength, our power.

1 Stand with your toes, ankles and knees together.

2 Lift your lower belly, draw your shoulders away from your ears and let your arms hang by your sides, palms facing forwards, fingers spread wide.

3 Relax your jaw and soften your gaze to look straight ahead.

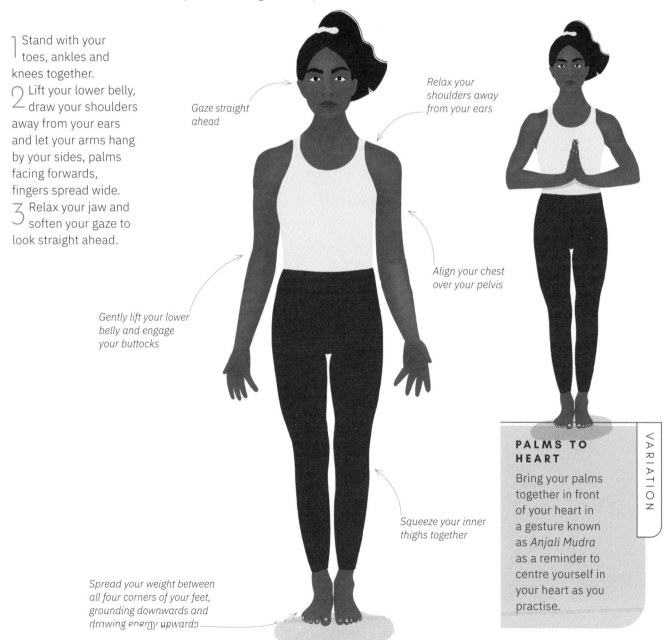

Gaze straight ahead

Relax your shoulders away from your ears

Align your chest over your pelvis

Gently lift your lower belly and engage your buttocks

Squeeze your inner thighs together

Spread your weight between all four corners of your feet, grounding downwards and drawing energy upwards

PALMS TO HEART

Bring your palms together in front of your heart in a gesture known as *Anjali Mudra* as a reminder to centre yourself in your heart as you practise.

VARIATION

Upward Salute

URDHVA HASTASANA

This pose gives us an experience of how important it is to build a strong foundation; how to root in order to rise.

1 Begin in Mountain Pose (*see* p. 64) and as you inhale, reach your arms overhead to bring your palms together.

2 Root yourself firmly to the ground through your feet and extend up through your spine, arms and fingertips.

3 Gently gaze towards your thumbs or the tip of your nose.

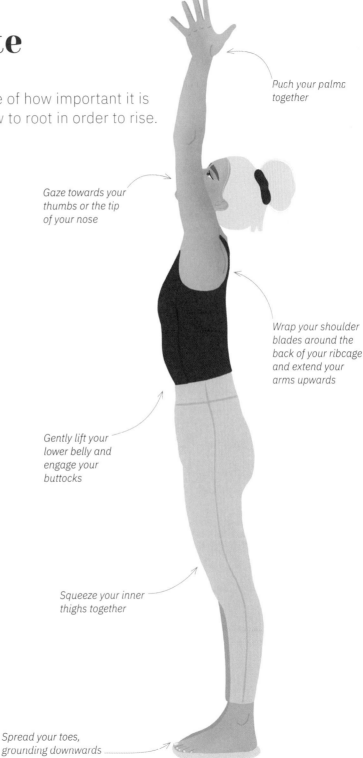

Puch your palms together

Gaze towards your thumbs or the tip of your nose

Wrap your shoulder blades around the back of your ribcage and extend your arms upwards

Gently lift your lower belly and engage your buttocks

Squeeze your inner thighs together

Spread your toes, grounding downwards

Standing Forward Bend
UTTANASANA

Forward bends require a delicate balance of strength and surrender. Focus on maintaining length in your spine while working with gravity to move deeper into the pose.

1 Stand with your feet hip-distance apart and align the outside edges of your feet so they are parallel.

2 Inhale as you bring your hands to your hips and lengthen your spine, drawing your energy upwards.

3 As you exhale, bow forwards, hinging from your hips to maintain the length in your spine.

4 Release your hands downwards to take hold of your shins, ankles or big toes if you can reach. You can keep your knees slightly bent if your hamstrings are particularly tight.

5 Gaze towards the tip of your nose and work with your breath so that on each inhalation there is a subtle lengthening of your spine and, on each exhalation, you gently draw yourself deeper into the pose.

6 To exit: Inhale and lengthen your spine, exhale and bring your hands to your hips and return to Mountain Pose (see p. 64) on your next inhale.

In the Sun Salutations (see pp. 58–61), you transition from Standing Forward Bend to either Half Forward Bend (see p. 67) or Upward Salute (see p. 65) so you do not need to exit via Mountain Pose here — only when the pose is practised in isolation.

TRANSITION NOTE

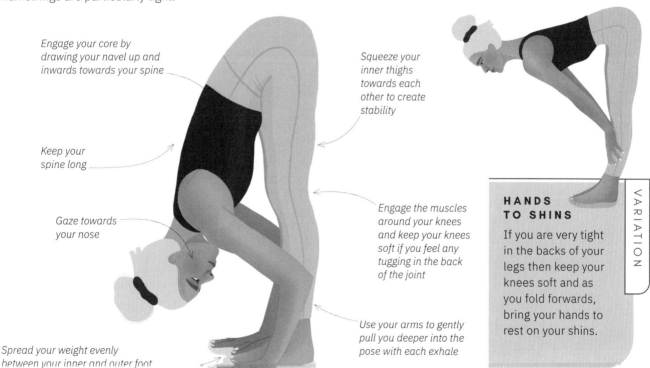

Engage your core by drawing your navel up and inwards towards your spine

Keep your spine long

Gaze towards your nose

Spread your weight evenly between your inner and outer foot

Squeeze your inner thighs towards each other to create stability

Engage the muscles around your knees and keep your knees soft if you feel any tugging in the back of the joint

Use your arms to gently pull you deeper into the pose with each exhale

HANDS TO SHINS

If you are very tight in the backs of your legs then keep your knees soft and as you fold forwards, bring your hands to rest on your shins.

VARIATION

Half Forward Bend

ARDHA UTTANASANA

This pose encourages a gentle lengthening in the spine to create space for a deeper forward fold.

1 From Standing Forward Bend (*see* p. 66), push your fingertips into the floor either just in front of you or beside your feet.

2 Inhale and straighten your elbows and lift your torso away from your thighs until your spine is parallel to the floor. If your hamstrings are tight, then raise your fingers on blocks.

3 Lengthen your breastbone forwards to create a subtle arch in your spine, softening your knees if you need to. Gaze towards your third eye in the middle of your forehead.

In the Sun Salutations (*see* pp. 58–61), you transition from Half Forward Bend to Plank Pose (*see* p. 68) by planting your hands in front of your feet and stepping or floating back.

TRANSITION NOTE

Create a slight arch in your spine

Gaze towards your third eye

Lift your heart and extend your breastbone forwards

Create as much space as possible between your pubic bone and your navel

Spread your weight evenly between your inner and outer foot

Push your fingertips into the floor

Plank Pose

PHALAKASANA

This pose helps to build core stability and upper body strength. If you notice any pain in your back, or if your hips start to sag, drop your knees to the ground.

1 Begin on your hands and knees with your shoulders stacked over your wrists and your index fingers pointing directly ahead of you. One at a time, step your feet back and straighten your legs.

2 Push the floor away through your hands and broaden your shoulder blades. Extend back through your heels and pull up on your kneecaps to activate your legs.

3 Lengthen your tailbone towards your heels and lift gently through your lower belly to create a straight line from the crown of your head back through your heels. Gaze downwards between your thumbs or to the tip of your nose.

In a Sun Salutation, you transition through Plank Pose as you move from Half Forward Bend (*see* p.67) to Four-limbed Staff Pose (*see* p. 69). Simply step or float back from Half Forward Bend into Plank Pose, bringing your knees to the ground if you need to.

TRANSITION NOTE

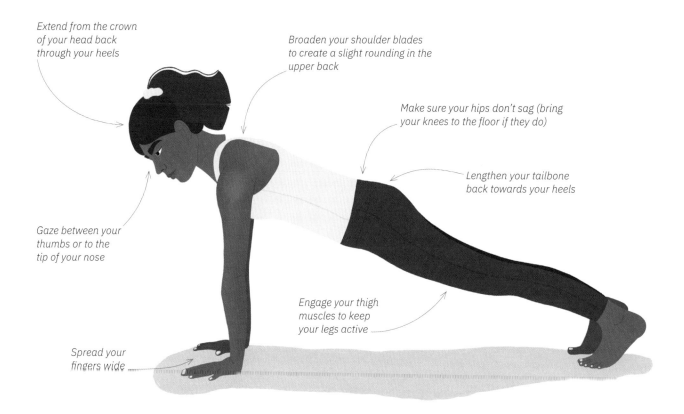

Extend from the crown of your head back through your heels

Broaden your shoulder blades to create a slight rounding in the upper back

Make sure your hips don't sag (bring your knees to the floor if they do)

Lengthen your tailbone back towards your heels

Gaze between your thumbs or to the tip of your nose

Engage your thigh muscles to keep your legs active

Spread your fingers wide

Four-limbed Staff Pose

CHATURANGA DANDASANA

This is a challenging pose that requires both mental and physical strength. If you feel you are losing the integrity of the pose in your Sun Salutations, either lower yourself all the way down to the ground or modify it with the variation below.

1 From Plank Pose (*see* p. 68), shift your weight into your hands and, on an exhalation, bend your elbows in towards your sides, lowering yourself downwards until your elbows are at right angles and you are hovering just above the ground.

2 Draw your shoulders back and down and keep your legs active, your chest open and your neck and spine parallel to the ground.

3 Gaze to the tip of your nose, bringing your knees to the ground if you find the full pose too intense.

In a Sun Salutation, you transition from Four-limbed Staff Pose (*see* p. 69) to Upward Dog (*see* p. 70) by pushing through your toes and lifting your chest. You can also hold Four-limbed Staff Pose as a way to build upper body and core strength so simply lower to the ground after a couple of breaths if you are practising this.

TRANSITION NOTE

KNEES TO FLOOR

Most people need to build strength before practising the full pose. Start in Plank Pose, lower your knees to the floor and as slowly as you can, bend your elbows and hover with your chest parallel to the floor for a few breaths before lowering all the way down.

VARIATION

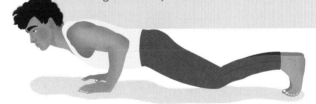

Draw your shoulders away from your ears

Keep your spine parallel to the floor

Firm your buttocks and lengthen your tailbone towards your heels

Pull up on your kneecaps to keep your legs active or drop your knees to the floor if it feels too intense

Gaze towards the tip of your nose

Hug your elbows into your waist

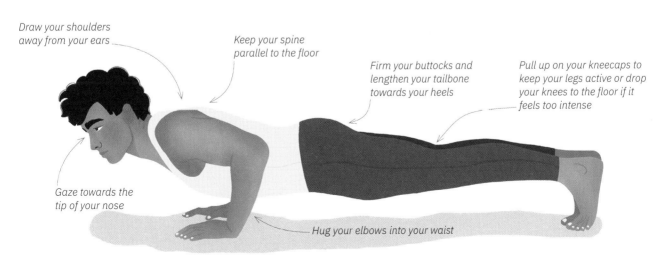

Upward Dog

URDHVA MUKHA SVANASANA

This is strong shape which requires spinal mobility and upper body strength. If you have any lower back pain then replace Upward Dog with Cobra Pose (*see* p. 71).

1 Lying on your front, slide your hands back so they are either side of your chest.

2 As you inhale, begin to lift your chest and extend through your spine as you straighten your arms, pushing the tops of your feet into the mat and lifting your thighs.

3 Root down firmly through your hands and extend your heart forwards. Lengthen your tailbone back towards your heels and lift your pubic bone to create an even curve throughout your spine and prevent dumping into the lower back.

4 Either gaze towards your third eye in the centre of your forehead or straight ahead.

5 To exit: Either lower back down to the floor or lift your hips and roll over your toes to Downward Dog (*see* p. 72).

Sun Salutations involve a transition from Four-limbed Staff Pose (*see* p.69) to Upward Dog. This is a challenging transition that requires you to push back through your toes to give you the forward momentum to lift your chest forwards and upwards. Feel free to drop your knees to the ground here or lower down on to your stomach before lifting to Upward Dog.

TRANSITION NOTE

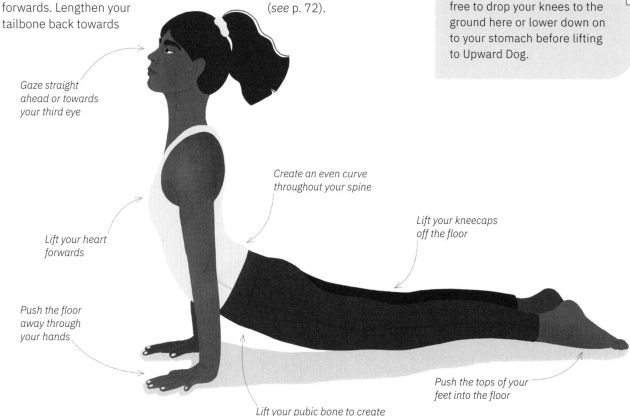

Gaze straight ahead or towards your third eye

Lift your heart forwards

Push the floor away through your hands

Create an even curve throughout your spine

Lift your kneecaps off the floor

Push the tops of your feet into the floor

Lift your pubic bone to create space in your lower back

Cobra Pose

BHUJANGASANA

This is a gentle backbend that works nicely as a preparatory pose for Upward Dog (*see* p. 70).

1 Lying on your front, place your hands underneath your shoulders. With your feet hip-distance apart, lengthen your tailbone towards your heels and lightly contract your buttocks.

2 As you inhale, push your hands firmly into the floor and lift your chest until a point where it feels good. Keep your arms bent and forearms on the floor if you need to and focus on creating an even curve throughout your entire spine instead of striving for a deep backbend. Gaze straight ahead or towards your third eye.

3 To exit: Lower back down onto your belly.

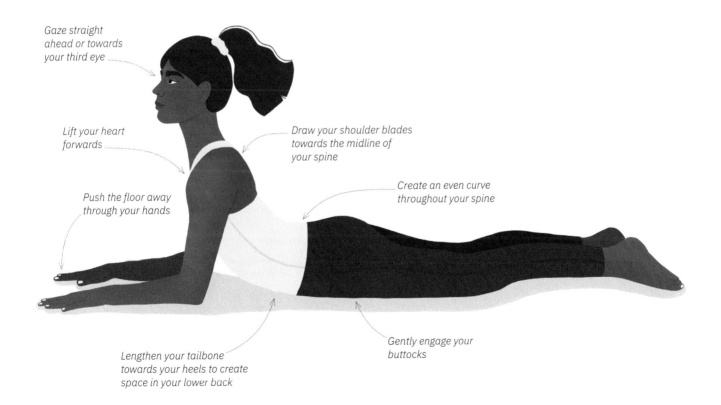

Gaze straight ahead or towards your third eye

Lift your heart forwards

Push the floor away through your hands

Draw your shoulder blades towards the midline of your spine

Create an even curve throughout your spine

Lengthen your tailbone towards your heels to create space in your lower back

Gently engage your buttocks

Downward Dog

ADHO MUKHA SVANASANA

This pose is a foundational pose that you will come across in almost all sequences and styles of yoga. It is both an inversion and an arm balance, as well as offering a stretch to the backs of your legs.

1 Begin on your hands and knees with your shoulders stacked over your wrists and index fingers pointing forwards. Hook your toes under and start straightening your legs to lift your sitting bones to the sky. As you do this, push your chest back towards your thighs to create an upturned V-shape. You can keep your knees slightly bent if you're particularly tight in the backs of your legs.

2 Push your hands firmly into the ground and lengthen through your spine, engaging a subtle *Uddiyana Bandha* (*see* p. 50) if you can.

3 Wrap your shoulder blades around the back of your rib cage to create space and stability. Let your head hang loosely and gaze towards the tip of your nose.

4 To exit: Drop your knees to the floor or step or float forwards to a Standing Forward Bend (*see* p. 66) if you are practising Downward Dog as part of a Sun Salutation.

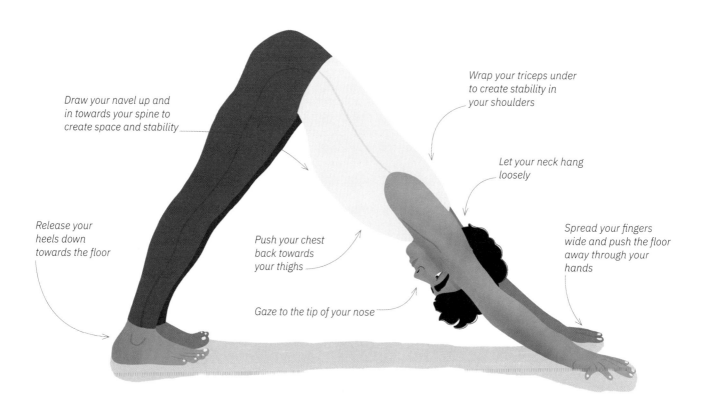

Draw your navel up and in towards your spine to create space and stability

Wrap your triceps under to create stability in your shoulders

Let your neck hang loosely

Release your heels down towards the floor

Push your chest back towards your thighs

Spread your fingers wide and push the floor away through your hands

Gaze to the tip of your nose

Chair Pose

UTKATASANA

This pose gives us a sense of rooting and rising, grounding and stretching, stability and openness.

1 Begin standing with your toes, ankles and knees together. Root down through all four corners of your feet, bend your knees and drop your hips until you can touch the floor either side of you with your fingertips. On an inhalation, sweep your arms forwards and overhead.

2 Push your palms together and gaze up towards your thumbs or towards your third eye. If it feels too intense to have your palms touching, then bring your hands shoulder-width apart or release your arms from overhead and bring your hands to rest on your thighs.

3 Lengthen your tailbone towards your heels, energising the deep layers of muscles either side of your spine and in your abdominals.

4 To exit: Straighten your legs and return to Mountain Pose (see p. 64).

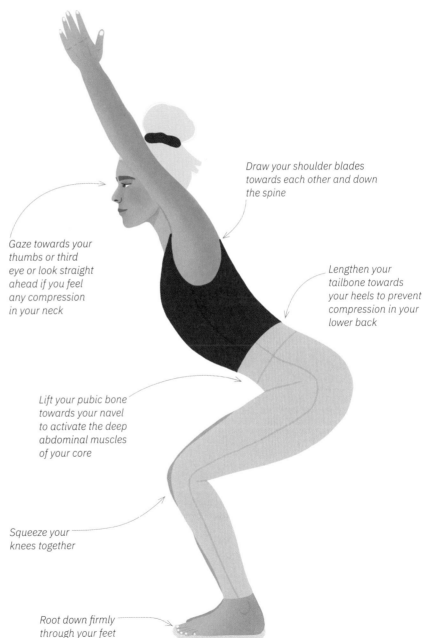

Draw your shoulder blades towards each other and down the spine

Gaze towards your thumbs or third eye or look straight ahead if you feel any compression in your neck

Lengthen your tailbone towards your heels to prevent compression in your lower back

Lift your pubic bone towards your navel to activate the deep abdominal muscles of your core

Squeeze your knees together

Root down firmly through your feet

Warrior One
VIRABHADRASANA A

Warrior One builds strength and stability as well as creating a sense of grounding and expansion.

1 From Mountain Pose (*see* p. 64) take a big step backwards with your left leg, turning your left toes out to a 45-degree angle.

2 Draw back on your right hip slightly and slide your left hip forwards to help square the hips and bend your right knee until your right thigh is parallel to the floor. Root down into the outside edge of your left foot to keep your left leg active.

3 Reach your hands up towards the sky, push your palms together and gaze towards your thumbs or third eye, creating a sense of lift and expansion throughout your whole body.

4 Align your shoulders over your chest and your chest over your pelvis. Lengthen your tailbone towards the floor to prevent compression in your lower back and sink down into the pose. If you notice your hips rotating outwards, lift your left heel to come onto the ball of your foot and square your hips.

5 To exit: Either step forwards to Mountain Pose (*see* p. 64) or, if practising as part of Sun Salutation B (*see* pp. 60–1, bring your hands to the floor and step back to Plank (*see* p. 68) before repeating on the other side.

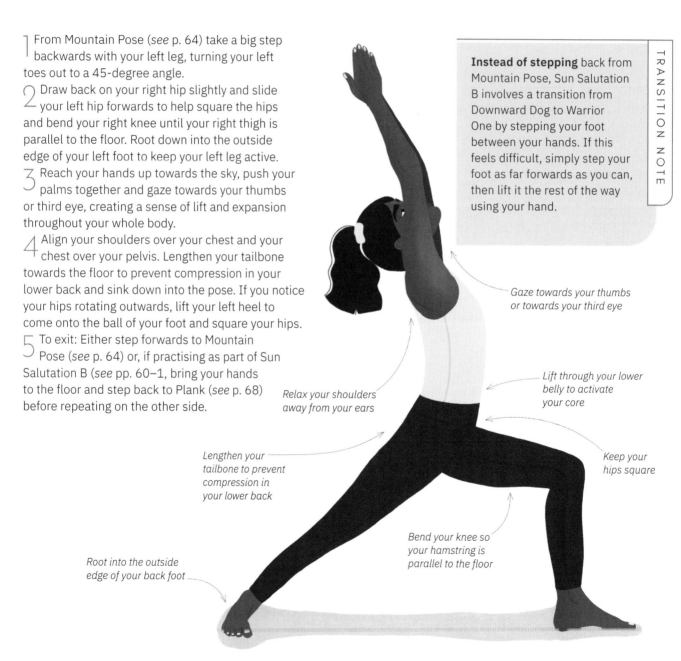

TRANSITION NOTE

Instead of stepping back from Mountain Pose, Sun Salutation B involves a transition from Downward Dog to Warrior One by stepping your foot between your hands. If this feels difficult, simply step your foot as far forwards as you can, then lift it the rest of the way using your hand.

Gaze towards your thumbs or towards your third eye

Relax your shoulders away from your ears

Lift through your lower belly to activate your core

Keep your hips square

Lengthen your tailbone to prevent compression in your lower back

Bend your knee so your hamstring is parallel to the floor

Root into the outside edge of your back foot

The Closing Sequence

The closing sequence brings balance to the dynamic nature of the rest of our practice. It calms us, grounds us and gives us an opportunity to fully absorb the benefits of our practice before we return to the demands of the outside world.

The closing sequence consists of three parts: an inversion, a simple seated pose that gives us space to draw our awareness inwards to our breath and Corpse Pose – our final relaxation. You might find it helpful to set a timer before you begin Corpse Pose so that you can fully relax without worrying about how long you've been in the pose.

1 **Shoulder Stand** (*see p. 77*), **Plough Pose** (*see p.78*) or **Legs Up the Wall Pose** (*see p. 79*), 10–25 breaths

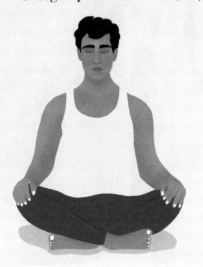

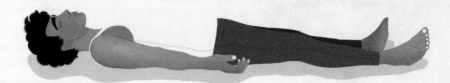

2 **Easy Pose** (*see p. 80*), 25 breaths

3 **Corpse Pose** (*see p. 81*), 5–10 minutes

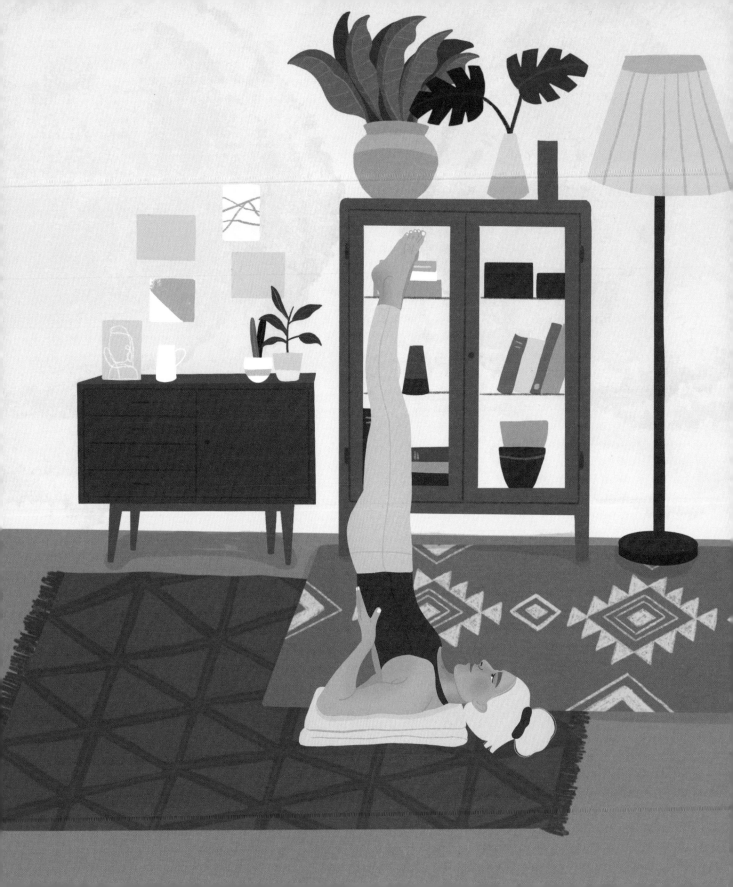

Shoulder Stand

SALAMBA SARVANGASANA

This is a beautiful inversion to finish your practice and it can be very calming if you are going through a moment of anxiety. If you have any neck issues, replace it with Legs Up the Wall Pose (*see* p.79).

1 Lying on your back with your knees bent and your hands palm downwards either side of you, push into your hands and lift your legs, curling up your spine to bring your knees towards your forehead.

2 Taking your weight in your shoulders and upper arms, position your hands on your lower back, drawing your shoulder blades towards each other to prevent your elbows winging out to the sides.

3 Mindfully begin to straighten your legs towards the sky so they are perpendicular to the floor. Stack your feet over your hips and your hips over your shoulders.

4 Create length in the back of your neck, avoiding over-tucking the chin, and gaze towards your navel.

5 To exit: Keeping your core engaged and with your hands supporting your back, slowly lower yourself back down to the floor, allowing your legs to come over your head to begin with, if need be.

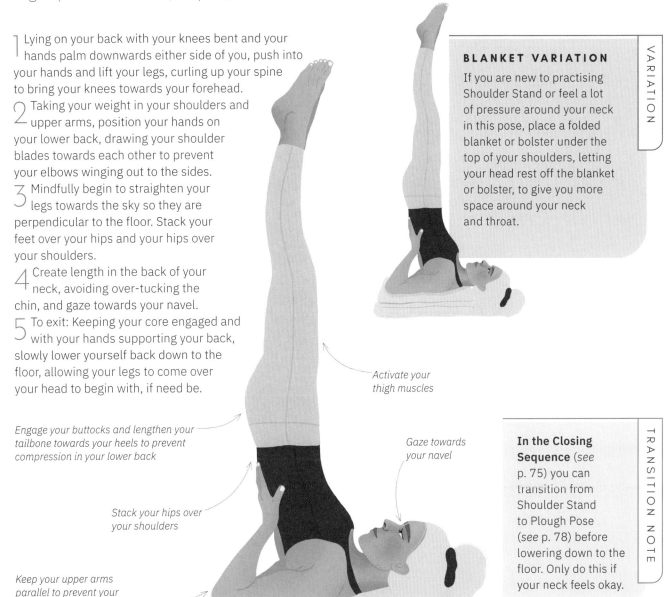

VARIATION

BLANKET VARIATION

If you are new to practising Shoulder Stand or feel a lot of pressure around your neck in this pose, place a folded blanket or bolster under the top of your shoulders, letting your head rest off the blanket or bolster, to give you more space around your neck and throat.

Activate your thigh muscles

Engage your buttocks and lengthen your tailbone towards your heels to prevent compression in your lower back

Gaze towards your navel

Stack your hips over your shoulders

Keep your upper arms parallel to prevent your elbows winging out

Draw your shoulder blades down your back

TRANSITION NOTE

In the Closing Sequence (*see* p. 75) you can transition from Shoulder Stand to Plough Pose (*see* p. 78) before lowering down to the floor. Only do this if your neck feels okay.

Plough Pose

HALASANA

Plough pose provides a gentle stretch to the entire back of the body while being calming to the nervous system. Traditionally, it's practised after Shoulder Stand (*see* p. 77). If you have any neck issues, Legs Up the Wall Pose (*see* p.79) is a beautiful alternative.

1 Lying on your back with your knees bent and your hands palms downwards either side of you, push into your hands and lift your legs, curling up your spine to bring your knees towards your forehead.

2 Taking your weight in your shoulders and upper arms, position your hands on your lower back, drawing your shoulder blades towards each other to prevent your elbows winging out to the sides.

3 Begin to straighten your legs towards the floor above your head, letting your toes rest on the ground if they reach (you can always place a bolster overhead if they don't reach). Point your toes, lengthen your chin away from your breast bone and gaze towards your navel.

4 To exit: Keeping your core engaged and with your hands supporting your back, slowly lower yourself back down to the floor.

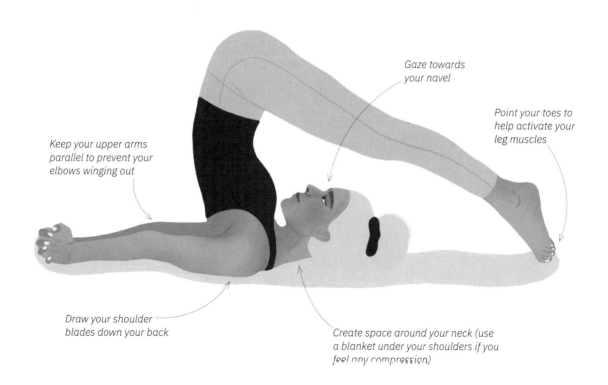

Gaze towards your navel

Point your toes to help activate your leg muscles

Keep your upper arms parallel to prevent your elbows winging out

Draw your shoulder blades down your back

Create space around your neck (use a blanket under your shoulders if you feel any compression)

Legs Up the Wall Pose

VIPARITA KARANI

This pose is a gentler alternative to Shoulder Stand (*see* p.77). It is my go-to pose for when I'm feeling anxious, exhausted or overwhelmed.

1 Sit sideways against a wall and swivel your legs around so you are lying on your back with your legs up against the wall, so that your torso and legs form an L-shape.

2 Relax into the wall and bring your hands to rest on your stomach or spread your arms wide either side of you, noticing if you are holding any tension in your upper body or face. Relax these areas too, if you are.

3 Close your eyes and allow yourself to release your weight into the floor beneath you. Feel free to play around with different props and variations. Raising your hips on a blanket feels lovely, and bending your legs and drawing your knees towards your chest can bring relief to aches and niggles in your lower back.

4 To exit: Wiggle yourself back away from the wall slightly and either make your way into Corpse Pose (*see* p. 81) or hug your knees into your chest, roll over to your side and push yourself back up to seated.

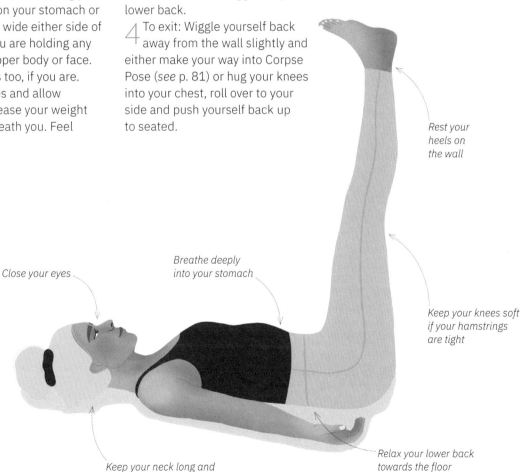

Rest your heels on the wall

Keep your knees soft if your hamstrings are tight

Close your eyes

Breathe deeply into your stomach

Relax your lower back towards the floor

Keep your neck long and your jaw relaxed

Easy Pose

SUKHASANA

Easy pose is a traditional position for breathwork and meditation. If you're used to sitting in chairs and rarely sit on the floor, it can be quite challenging to begin with so be patient as your hips open and your core strengthens.

1 Sit on the front of your sitting bones with your legs crossed at the shins, your knees wide and each foot under the opposite knee, keeping a comfortable gap between your feet and your pelvis. Gently flex your feet (pull your toes backwards towards your shins) to ensure you are rotating from your hip socket instead of your knee.

2 Grounding your tailbone towards the floor, extend your spine so your shoulders and ribcage are stacked over the bowl of your pelvis. Draw your shoulder blades down your spine towards the midline and lift your heart forwards, drawing your lower front ribs downwards to prevent overarching your back.

3 Rest your hands on your thighs, relax your shoulders and either gaze straight ahead or close your eyes.

SUPPORTED VARIATIONS

If you feel as though you are about to roll backwards, either place a folded blanket underneath your bottom or lean against a wall to give you extra support. If you feel any knee pain in this pose, come out gently and either sit on a chair or practise Staff Pose (*see* p. 133) instead.

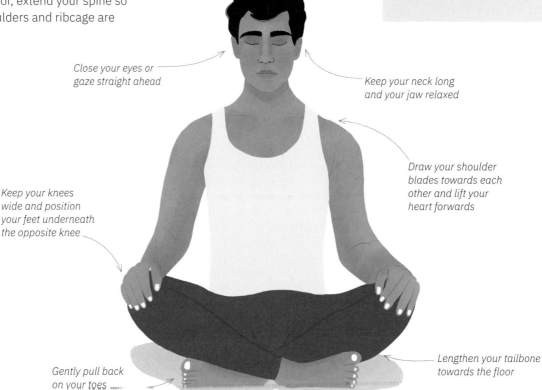

Close your eyes or gaze straight ahead

Keep your neck long and your jaw relaxed

Draw your shoulder blades towards each other and lift your heart forwards

Keep your knees wide and position your feet underneath the opposite knee

Lengthen your tailbone towards the floor

Gently pull back on your toes

Corpse Pose

SAVASANA

Corpse Pose asks us to relax into our body, to totally surrender to the present moment without judgement and to let ourselves be held by the ground beneath us. I would encourage you to practise it for at least five minutes at the end of every self-practice.

1 Lying on your back, take a deep inhalation, stretch your arms above your head, point your toes and tense every muscle in your body.

2 As you exhale, release all this tension, bringing your arms down by your sides with your palms to the sky and letting your feet wing out about hip-distance apart.

3 Close your eyes, release any control over your breath and let yourself relax here. Feel free to use any blankets, bolsters and eye masks to make the pose more restorative.

BENT KNEE

If lying flat on your back feels uncomfortable, bend your knees and let them fall inwards to take any pressure off your lower back.

VARIATION

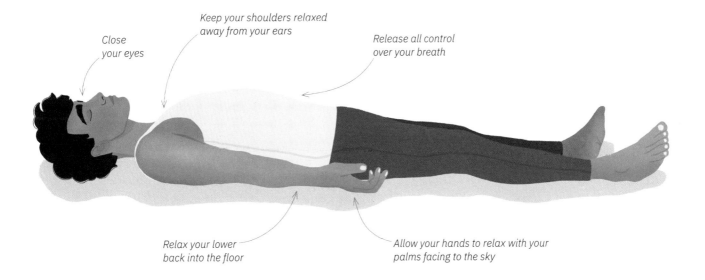

Close your eyes

Keep your shoulders relaxed away from your ears

Release all control over your breath

Relax your lower back into the floor

Allow your hands to relax with your palms facing to the sky

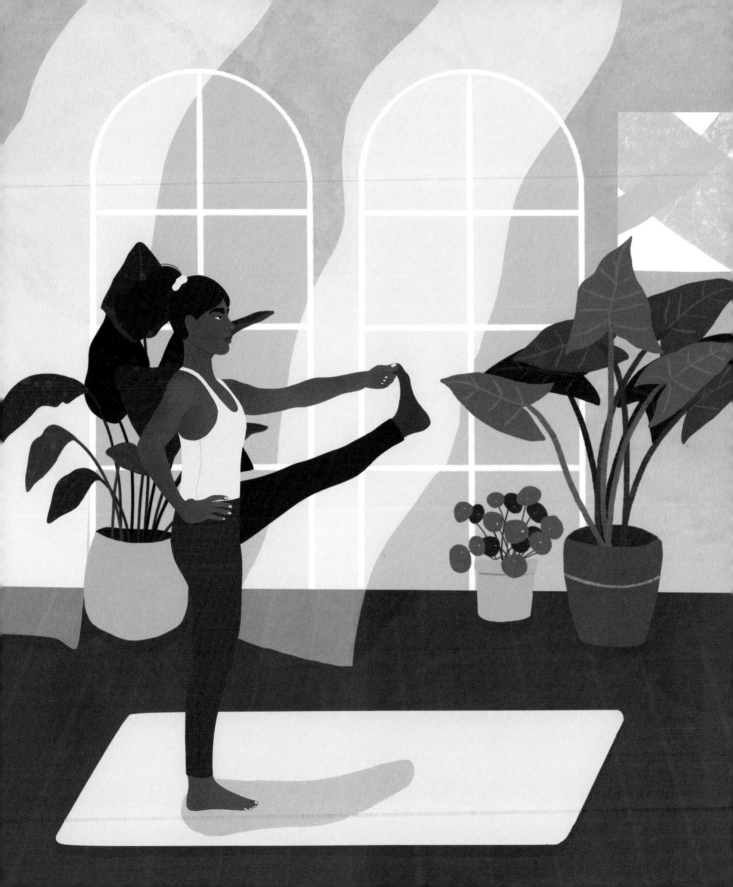

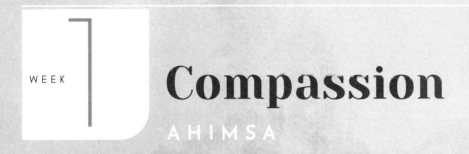

WEEK

1

Compassion

AHIMSA

THE JOURNEY OF YOGA is built upon a foundation of non-harm and compassion: *ahimsa*. The practice of non-harm must begin with ourselves. We must stop the war inside. We must welcome the parts of ourselves that are difficult to love. We must come face to face with our own pain and shame and unworthiness if we are to transform them into a loving force of compassion and kindness. Because until we stop harming ourselves – through thoughts, words and actions – and begin to hold ourselves with unconditional kindness, we will remain trapped by the conditioning of the society we are trying to transform. A society that profits from our subtle acts of self-harm and self-hate.

Accepting ourselves unconditionally – with all our mistakes and shadows and scars – is one of the most profound acts of non-harm we can practise. Sadly, many modern forms of yoga, as well as fitness classes, life coaching and even self-help books contain seeds of harm that encourage us to wage war against our imperfections. To fix ourselves. To become better, worthier, more acceptable. But, if we think we need fixing, we will keep looking for the broken places and become blind to our wholeness. To practise yoga is not about fixing ourselves but loving whatever is here. Because we never needed fixing. We were never broken. We were never damaged. We simply confused our humanness for brokenness. We have always been whole. And *ahimsa* is, quite often, the very first step on the path to realising this wholeness.

We harm ourselves in many ways. Some obvious, some subtle. Sometimes intentionally, sometimes automatically. Many acts of self-harm have become so normal for us that, until we truly look at ourselves and our lives, we don't realise we are causing ourselves

suffering at all: negative self-talk, putting everyone else's needs before our own, staying in destructive relationships, isolating ourselves, overeating, undereating, over-exercising, overworking, perfectionism, procrastination, not speaking up, not apologising, not forgiving, not letting go.

Ahimsa invites us to look at ourselves honestly to see where we are at war with our body, our relationships and our lives. It asks us to stop the war inside. Not just once, but over and over again. It calls us to practise non-harm in our daily life until kindness and compassion become our way of being.

Mindful Living Practice

Journal prompts

There is no exact formula for *ahimsa*. Unlearning the habit of self-harm is a unique journey for each of us. But it is always rooted in self-awareness – in understanding the ways in which we sabotage and betray ourselves – and in the tiny, daily practices that teach us that we are worthy of love and compassion. Use the questions below to explore where you may be causing harm to yourself and how you can practise *ahimsa*.

How am I causing harm to myself or others?

How can I practise non-harm in my daily life?

An example might be: 'I am causing harm to myself by eating for comfort when I am stressed. I can practise non-harm by noticing when I have the urge to overeat and, instead of acting on it, give myself space to feel the emotion and explore it through journalling.' Another example could be: 'I am causing harm to myself by always telling myself I am never good enough. I can practise non-harm by noticing my self-destructive thoughts instead of getting lost in them and consciously speaking to myself with kindness and gentleness.'

Aspiration inspiration

Aspirations – statements to aspire to – are powerful in opening us to a gentler, more compassionate way of being in the world. This week, see if you can create an aspiration that invites self-compassion into your life. For example:

'May I be loving and kind with myself.'

'May I see my worth and treat myself with respect and nourishment.'

'May I have the courage to look at myself honestly so I can see the ways I am causing myself to suffer. And may I have the compassion to treat myself with the same tenderness as someone I love deeply.'

It's worth noting that aspirations are slightly different to affirmations. Aspirations, which begin 'May I ...', invite change by opening us to a new way of being, whereas affirmations, which usually begin 'I am ...', force change upon us, as though we are trying to convince ourselves that we are someone we are not, often creating inner resistance. Telling ourselves, 'I am beautiful' (especially if we don't believe it) feels very different to the openness of: 'May I see the beauty within me.' Aspirations allow us to accept ourselves as we are while creating space for love, peace and compassion to grow.

RAINDROPs of compassion

This is a beautiful practice that helps us to cultivate compassion for ourselves and gives us a framework to work with when we experience challenging emotions. The original practice is really summed up in the acronym RAIN:

- **R**ecognise – What is actually happening? What thoughts, feelings, behaviours and physical sensations am I experiencing right now?
- **A**llow – Can I allow those thoughts, feelings and sensations to simply be there? Can I accept whatever is arising without trying to numb, fix or avoid it?
- **I**nvestigate (without judgement) – How does this experience feel in my body? What is asking for my attention?
- **N**urture – What do I need right now? Sleep, space, stillness, connection, nature, reassurance? What would be the kindest and most loving thing I could do for myself right now?

To deepen this practice, we can begin to explore our conditioned defences: the way we close our hearts, distract ourselves and resist our experiences. By exploring these patterns with curiosity and compassion – instead of judgement and shame – these defences become gateways to our freedom. The acronym DROP gives us a framework to do this:

- **D**istraction – How am I distracting myself from my feelings and experiences?
- **R**esistance – How am I resisting reality?
- **O**bliviousness – How am I ignoring what I am experiencing? What am I suppressing?
- **P**unishment – How am I judging or punishing myself for what I am experiencing?

You can begin to practise RAINDROPs through journalling and, as you become more fluent in the practice, see if you can use it when you notice yourself feeling stressed or overwhelmed throughout your day. If you would like to learn more, I would highly recommend the teachings of mindfulness teacher, Michele McDonald (who first coined the term RAIN) and Tara Brach who has developed the practice further.

Breathwork – *pranayama*

This week, if you haven't already, begin introducing Victorious Breath (*see* p. 63) into your *asana* practice, moving with your breath while slightly restricting the back of your throat to create internal heat. You might find it helpful to practise Victorious Breath for a few minutes in a comfortable seated position before you begin your *asana* practise. If you find that it makes you feel dizzy or your breath becomes strained, simply focus on breathing steadily and rhythmically using Equal Breathing (see p. 62) and introduce Victorious Breath into your practice again in a couple of weeks.

Meditation

Exhalation-counting Meditation

When we begin meditating, we often assume that 10 minutes of meditation can undo 10 years of anxiety. That it will take away all our stress and fill us with peace. In reality, meditation is about welcoming whatever shows up – grief, pain, fear, joy, love, regret – instead of fighting it. It gives us the space to heal the violence within us.

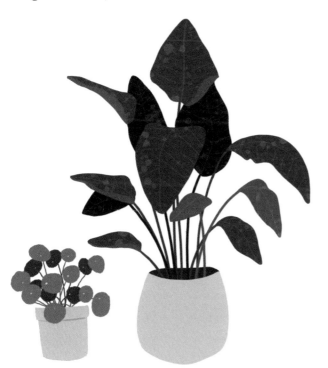

To stop the war inside. To focus on our habits, patterns and conditioning so that, as the *Yoga Sutras* say, we can 'gain knowledge and understanding of our past and of how we can change the patterns that aren't serving us to live more freely and fully'.

The first thing we have to learn in meditation is how to be still. How to step away from the world and its constant need for busyness. As we find physical stillness, our mind begins to settle into stillness too. But sitting still – without fidgeting or wriggling, or scratching that itch – is often quite challenging so take some time to find a comfortable seated position where you feel relaxed and aware and then return to this posture each time you meditate. Many people find Easy Pose (*see* p. 80) good for meditation, but find a position that feels comfortable for you. Feel free to kneel, use props and cushion, rest against a wall or sit on a chair.

This week, use a simple exhalation-counting meditation to train your mind in how to pay attention to a single object: your breath. Find a comfortable seated position, close your eyes and let your mind and body settle. Bring your awareness to your breath and as you exhale, silently say 'one'. On your next exhale, say 'two', and so on until you reach ten and then begin again from one. Try not to control your breath, simply be aware of it.

It's likely that after a few breaths your mind will wander to something else: what you're having for dinner tonight, that email you forgot to send, the pain in your shoulder. When this happens (which it will), simply notice that your mind has wandered, bring your awareness back to your breath and return to counting your exhalations, beginning at one.

This week, I'd recommend meditating for just two minutes a day so it's easy to squeeze in after your *asana* practice, first thing in the morning, or in the tiny spaces that open up in daily life. If you like, you might find it helpful to set a two-minute alarm before you begin your meditating so that you can be fully present without worrying about how long you've been practising. Equally, if you don't have to rush off anywhere, you might find that towards the end of the week you'd like to spend a bit more time meditating – maybe four or five minutes – so give yourself the freedom to meditate for longer if you feel called to do so.

Asanas: Standing Forward Bends

ALLOW 15–20 MINUTES

This week, introduce a series of standing forward bends to your practice. Simply practise the opening sequence, followed by the five new poses, and then finally the closing sequence. See if you can bring the intention of non-harm on to the mat with you, pulling back when you need to. Again, I'd recommend you practise this sequence until you can remember the new poses by heart before moving on to Week Two. You can find detailed instructions on each forward bend over the next few pages.

1 **Opening Sequence**

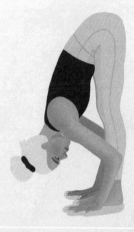

2 **Standing Forward Bend** (*see p. 66*), 5 breaths

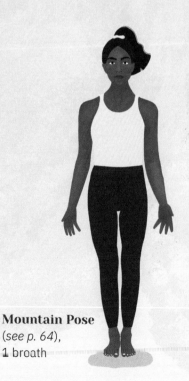

6 **Mountain Pose** (*see p. 64*), 1 breath

7 **Wide-legged Standing Forward Bend** (*see p. 90*), 5 breaths

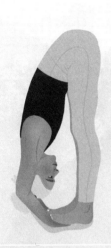

3 **Hand Under Foot Pose**
(*see p. 88*),
5 breaths

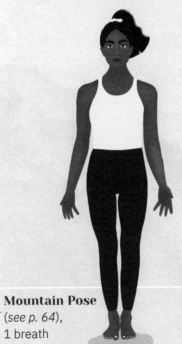

4 **Mountain Pose**
(*see p. 64*),
1 breath

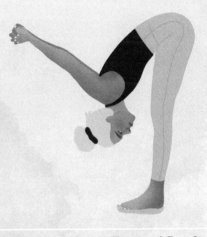

5 **Bound Hands Forward Bend**
(*see p. 89*),
5 breaths

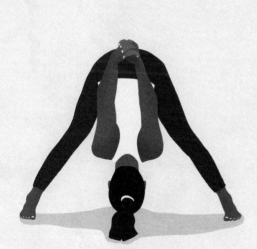

8 **Bound Hands Wide-legged**
Forward Bend (*see p. 91*),
5 breaths

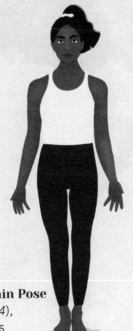

9 **Mountain Pose**
(*see p. 64*),
5 breaths

10 **Closing Sequence**

Hand Under Foot Pose

PADA HASTASANA

This is a deeper variation of Standing Forward Bend (*see* p. 66), so if it feels too intense, listen to your body and replace it with a Standing Forward Bend.

1 Stand with your feet hip-distance apart and align the outside edges of your feet so they are parallel.

2 Inhale as you bring your hands to your hips and lengthen your spine, drawing your energy upwards.

3 As you exhale, bow forwards, hinging from your hips to maintain the length in your spine.

4 Release your hands down to the floor, palms facing upwards, and, one at a time, step the ball of each foot onto each palm, distributing your weight evenly between all four corners of each foot.

5 Gaze towards the tip of your nose, draw your navel towards your spine, engaging *Uddiyana Bandha* (*see* p. 50), and work with your breath to gently draw yourself deeper into the pose on each exhale.

6 To exit: Inhale and lengthen your spine to Half Forward Bend (*see* p. 67), exhale, bringing your hands to your hips and inhale, standing up to Mountain Pose (*see* p. 64).

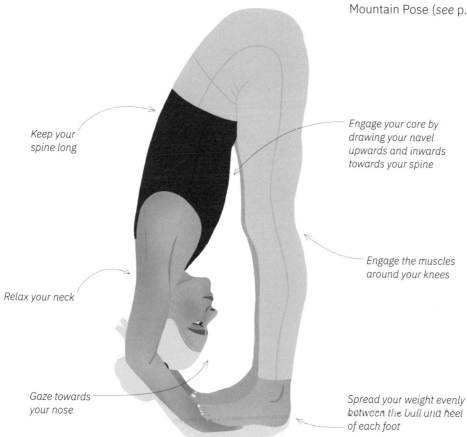

Keep your spine long

Engage your core by drawing your navel upwards and inwards towards your spine

Relax your neck

Engage the muscles around your knees

Gaze towards your nose

Spread your weight evenly between the ball and heel of each foot

Bound Hands Forward Bend

BADDHA HASTA UTTANASANA

This is a more active forward bend that creates openness across the shoulders and upper back while encouraging you to keep your spine long and your chest open.

1 Stand with your feet hip-distance apart and align the outside edges of your feet so they are parallel.

2 Interlace your fingers behind your back and, as you exhale, fold forwards, stretching your arms up and away from you.

3 Gaze towards the tip of your nose and work with your breath to gently bring your hands further over your head with each exhale.

4 To exit: Soften your knees and, on an inhale, slowly come back up to standing, releasing your hands to Mountain Pose (see p. 64).

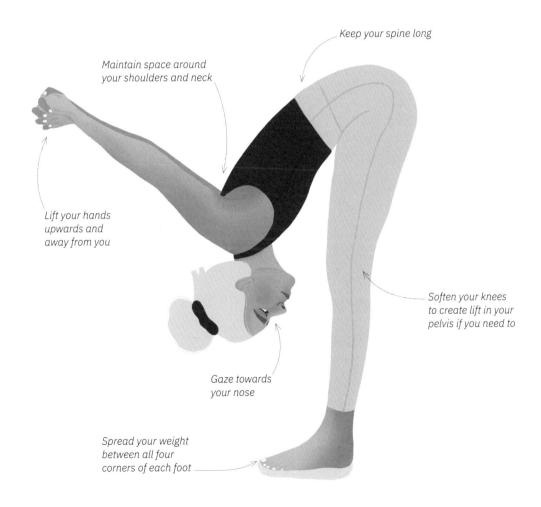

Maintain space around your shoulders and neck

Keep your spine long

Lift your hands upwards and away from you

Soften your knees to create lift in your pelvis if you need to

Gaze towards your nose

Spread your weight between all four corners of each foot

Wide-legged Standing Forward Bend

PRASARITA PADDOTTANASANA A

This pose provides a strong stretch for the muscles around the hips, backs of the legs and inner thighs. If you have low blood pressure, come out of this pose slowly.

1 From Mountain Pose (*see* p. 64), step your left foot back about one leg-length and rotate your hips so they are facing the long edge of your mat. Turn your toes inwards slightly.

2 Inhale as you bring your hands to your hips, lengthening your spine and drawing your energy upwards.

3 As you exhale, bow forwards, hinging from your hips. Release your hands downwards to the floor, shoulder-width apart with your fingers in line with your big toes and release the crown of your head towards the ground, gazing towards the tip of your nose.

4 Keep the pose active by lifting the inner arches of your feet and draw your navel towards your spine. Play around making your stance wider or narrower to create more stability or a stronger stretch.

5 To exit: Inhale and lengthen your spine to a wide-legged variation of Half Forward Bend (*see* p. 67). Exhale, bringing your hands to your hips and, on an inhale, lift your chest. Exhale and either transition to Bound Hands Wide-legged Forward Bend (*see* p. 91) or step your feet together in Mountain Pose (*see* p. 64).

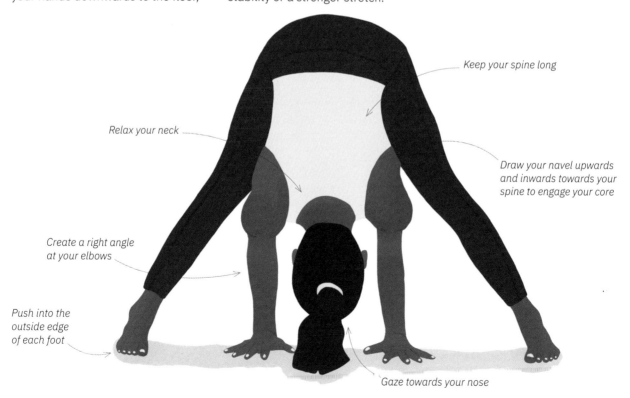

Keep your spine long

Relax your neck

Draw your navel upwards and inwards towards your spine to engage your core

Create a right angle at your elbows

Push into the outside edge of each foot

Gaze towards your nose

Bound Hands Wide-legged Forward Bend

BADDHA HASTA PRASARITA PADDOTTANASANA
(ALSO KNOWN AS) PRASARITA PADDOTTANASANA C

Interlacing your fingers adds another element to this pose, building both stability and openness.

1 From Mountain Pose (*see* p. 64), step your left foot back about one leg-length and rotate your hips so they are facing the long edge of your mat. Turn your toes inwards slightly.

2 Interlace your fingers behind your back and as you exhale, bow forwards, hinging from your hips, stretching your arms upwards and away from you and releasing the crown of your head towards the ground. Gaze towards the tip of your nose.

3 Keep your neck relaxed and with each exhale, gently lift your hands further overhead.

4 To exit: Soften your knees and, on an inhale, slowly come back up to standing, releasing your hands and stepping your feet together into Mountain Pose (*see* p. 64).

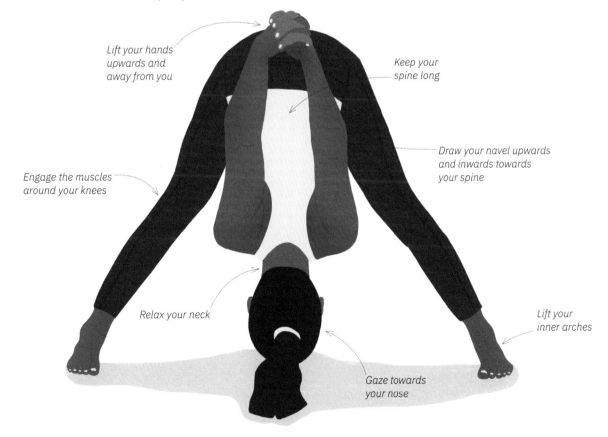

Lift your hands upwards and away from you

Keep your spine long

Engage the muscles around your knees

Draw your navel upwards and inwards towards your spine

Relax your neck

Lift your inner arches

Gaze towards your nose

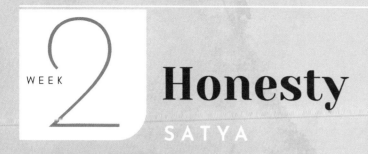

Honesty

SATYA

TRUTHFULNESS IS A BEAUTIFUL, and sometimes brutal, thing. To be honest with ourselves about who we are, rather than hiding behind a mask, gives us freedom. And to see other people exactly as they are, instead of how we wish they would be, gives them freedom.

This week focuses on the mindful living practice of *satya*, interpreted as 'non-lying', 'ultimate truth' and 'what is ultimately real'. *Satya* is about much more than simply not telling lies. It means being in the world as it is instead of living in a fantasy we've created in our heads, unlearning what is untrue, unhelpful and unnecessary, and becoming more and more of our true Self. But being true to ourselves isn't always easy, especially when there are so many voices in the world – parents, teachers, friends, the media and society – telling us who we should be.

Practising *satya* encourages us to recognise the masks we are wearing, the beliefs we have absorbed from society and the goals we are chasing that were never really our own. It asks us to begin peeling back the layers of everything we are not – cultural conditioning, outgrown identities, other people's expectations – so we can become more of who we are. It invites us to look at ourselves honestly: about where we are holding ourselves back, what subtle addictions trap us and what we need to let go of in order to live with more freedom.

Practising *satya* guides us to think, speak and act with integrity, from a place that is rooted in deep compassion. When we stop and reflect on whether we are being honest with ourselves and in our interactions, we are often shocked at how many times throughout the day we find ourselves lying or being inauthentic (on average, we tell ten lies a day!). This is usually out of fear

or a desire to protect someone we love rather than to intentionally deceive.

When we begin practising *satya*, we might catch ourselves making an excuse to a friend who has invited us over for dinner that we already have plans instead of simply saying we are exhausted and need an early night. Or we might realise that we keep saying we'll have an alcohol-free night tomorrow when we have no real intention of doing so. Or we might find ourselves caught in a cycle of self-judgement, treating the thoughts that whisper how we should be thinner or prettier or more successful as ultimate truths instead of as conditioning from the corporate, consumeristic culture we live in. If we are practising *satya*, instead of saying, 'My stomach is too fat', – which is a judgement – we might say a non-judgemental truth such as, 'My body does not meet the narrow and unattainable socially constructed standard of beauty.' Replacing our judgements with honest awareness allows us to loosen the tight grip we have on our thoughts and beliefs and open up to a more compassionate way of being in the world. By seeing ourselves and our lives honestly, we can begin to question the conditioned beliefs we have mistakenly thought of as truths: 'Where did I learn that my stomach is too fat? Who profits from me believing this? How would it feel to accept my body as it is while being open to how it might change as I invest time and energy in my health?'

In many ways, *satya* is about slowing down, waking up

and being mindful of the thoughts we think, words we say and actions we take. By asking ourselves, 'Is this true? Is this kind?', we can free ourselves from the beliefs that hurt us, release the habits that are holding us back and catch a glimpse of who we are beneath the masks we wear.

Mindful Living Practice

Journal prompts

Before we can be more honest, we need to recognise the ways in which we are not being truthful with ourselves or others. Use the journal questions below to help explore where you might be lying to yourself, how you could be judging yourself and what masks you are wearing.

'Where am I not being honest with myself or others?'

'When do I pretend to be someone I am not?'

'How can I practise honesty in my daily life?'

For example, as we journal, we might discover: 'I am not being honest with my partner about my needs and how managing the household responsibilities on my own is leaving me feeling resentful.' Identifying where we are not speaking our truth allows us to explore ways in which we can begin practising honesty in our daily life: 'I can practise honesty by spending at least five minutes a day sharing how I feel and what I need with my partner and allowing them space to do the same.'

Aspiration inspiration

Use the ideas below to inspire you to create a daily aspiration that will invite more honesty into your life.

'May I have the courage to meet life unmasked.'

'May I be able to tell the difference between what I have been taught to believe and what is true.'

'May I live in alignment with my values.'

Discovering your values

When we have spent a lot of our life disconnected from our true Self, we often lose touch with our values and what is really important to us. By identifying what our true values are, we can take an honest stock of our lives and our goals and notice where we might be living out of alignment with them. Use the list below to inspire you to reflect on your values so you can live in a way that feels more authentic, more honest, more true.

Acceptance, achievement, ambition, awareness, balance, beauty, bravery, calmness, community, compassion, consciousness, contribution, courage, creativity, dependability, discipline, empathy, enthusiasm, ethical living, fame, family, freedom, friendship, generosity, grace, gratitude, hard work, health, hope, independence, intuition, justice, kindness, logic, love, loyalty, motivation, openness, optimism, passion, peace, playfulness, power, presence, purpose, respect, selflessness, sensitivity, service, spirituality, status, success, thoughtfulness, trustworthiness, vitality, wealth, wisdom.

Meditation

Inhalation-counting Meditation

Meditation offers us the opportunity to meet ourselves unmasked – often for the first time. By paying attention – to our breath, the sensations in our body, the present moment – we begin to experience ourselves, our lives and the world in a more honest, more naked way without our conditioning, prejudices and bias.

For this week's meditation practice, instead of counting your exhalations, count each inhalation from one to ten, beginning at one again each time your mind wanders. In the same way it takes time to build physical strength, it takes time to strengthen the mind; to learn to focus and maintain our awareness on a single object of attention (in this case, our inhalation). So, if you notice that every time you try to focus on your breath a thousand thoughts jump into your mind – hopes, worries, memories – be gentle with yourself. Most people can focus on their breath for only five to 30 seconds when they begin meditating. As your meditation practice becomes more consistent, your mind will wander less often and you will be able to bring it back far more quickly when it does.

If you have time this week, you might want to explore increasing your meditation practice to five to ten minutes.

Asanas: Leg-strengthening Poses

ALLOW 20-25 MINUTES

This week, we introduce four new poses: our warrior series. These are strong poses that can be challenging to begin with. Bringing *satya* into our practice allows us to be honest with ourselves about how deep we can go into a pose and how intensely we can practise that day. Sometimes we have a strong, dynamic practice planned, but when we step on the mat, we feel exhausted. If this happens, be honest with yourself and choose a gentler practice like the calming sequence in Part Three (*see* p. 176).

If you're struggling with a pose, notice what your mind is saying. If your thoughts are screaming, 'I am so rubbish at yoga', look for the truth instead: 'I'm finding this posture challenging right now.' Our time on the mat is a beautiful opportunity to discover what is true and how we can live from that place of truth within us.

1 **Opening Sequence** (*p. 58*)

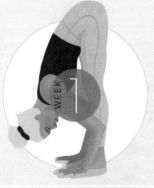

2 Repeat **WEEK ONE: Standing Forward Bends** (this is the sequence from last week — *see pp. 86–7* for a reminder)

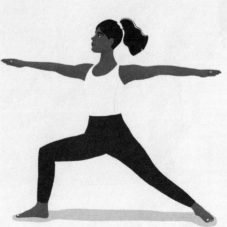

6 **Warrior Two** (*see p. 97*), 5 breaths then transition to next pose

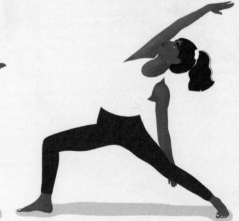

7 **Reverse Warrior** (*see p. 98*), 5 breaths then transition to next pose.

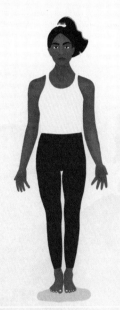

3 **Mountain Pose**
(*see p. 64*)

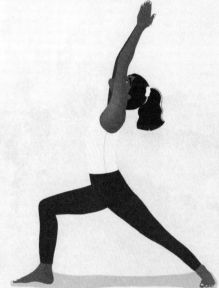

4 **Warrior One**
(*see p. 74*), 5 breaths then
transition to next pose

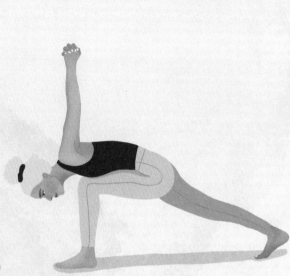

5 **Humble Warrior**
(*see p. 96*), 5 breaths then
transition to next pose

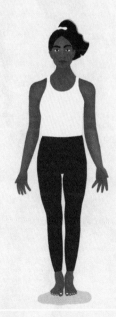

8 **Mountain Pose,**
5 breaths

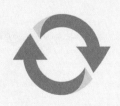

9 **Repeat poses**
4–8 on other side

10 **Closing Sequence**
(*see p. 75*)

PRACTICE REMINDER

'**Transition to next pose**' means to move from one pose to the next in a mini-sequence before repeating the same mini-sequence on the left side.

Humble Warrior

BADDHA VIRABHADRASANA

This pose requires a balance of power and humility, teaching us the strength required to surrender.

1 From Warrior One (*see* p. 74) release your hands behind your back and interlace your fingers.

2 Ground yourself by distributing your weight between both feet and, as you exhale, bow forwards, lifting your hands upwards and away from you. Either rest your chest on your thigh, or if your body feels open enough, bow your head towards the inside of your front foot, keeping your hips facing forwards.

3 Relax your neck and gaze to the tip of your nose.

4 To exit: Inhale, slowly lift your chest, releasing your hands from behind your back and reaching overhead back to Warrior One.

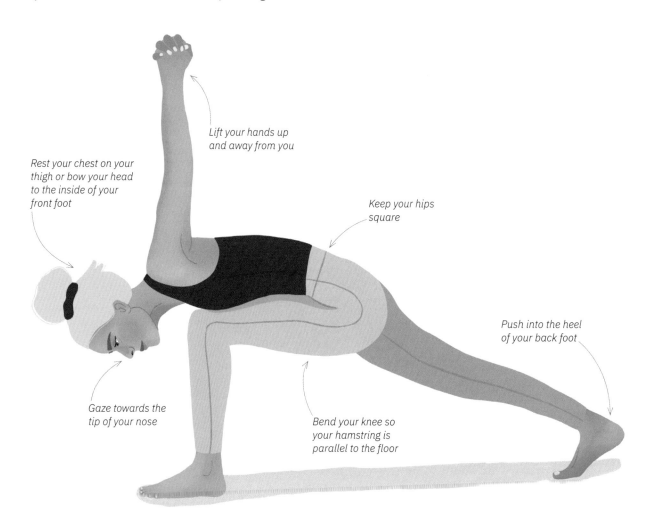

Lift your hands up and away from you

Rest your chest on your thigh or bow your head to the inside of your front foot

Keep your hips square

Push into the heel of your back foot

Gaze towards the tip of your nose

Bend your knee so your hamstring is parallel to the floor

Warrior Two

VIRABHADRASANA B

This pose cultivates strength, openness and focus, drawing your awareness inwards to help you reinhabit your body.

1 From Warrior One (*see* p. 74), keeping your feet and legs in the same place, rotate through your hips so that you are facing the long edge of your mat and reach your arms out wide.

2 Refine the pose by lengthening your tailbone towards the floor, gently lifting through the pubic bone and relaxing your shoulders. Be mindful that your front knee doesn't fall inwards by activating your gluteal muscles. Gaze over the middle finger of your front hand.

3 To exit: Depending on the pose you are transitioning to, either lean back to Reverse Warrior (*see* p. 98), step your feet together into Mountain Pose (*see* p. 64) or take your palms to the mat either side of your front foot and step back into Downward Dog (*see* p. 72).

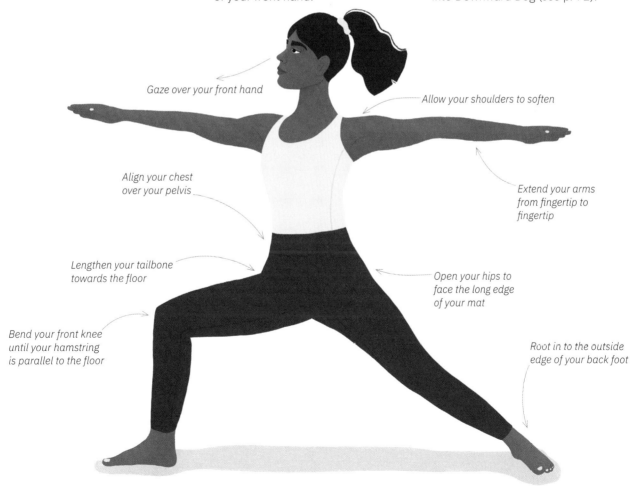

Gaze over your front hand

Allow your shoulders to soften

Align your chest over your pelvis

Extend your arms from fingertip to fingertip

Lengthen your tailbone towards the floor

Open your hips to face the long edge of your mat

Bend your front knee until your hamstring is parallel to the floor

Root in to the outside edge of your back foot

Reverse Warrior

VIPARITA VIRABHADRASANA

Reverse Warrior brings a deep stretch into the side body and encourages us to find strength from the ground up.

1 From Warrior Two (*see* p. 97), with your right foot forwards, spin your right palm upwards to face the sky. Inhale and, lengthening up through the crown of your head, lean backwards to bring your left hand to rest on your back leg. Your right arm will naturally extend overhead.

2 Keep rooted through your feet, maintain the length in the underside of your body (remember that deeper does not mean better) and gaze towards the fingers of your right hand.

3 To exit: On an inhale, return to Warrior Two.

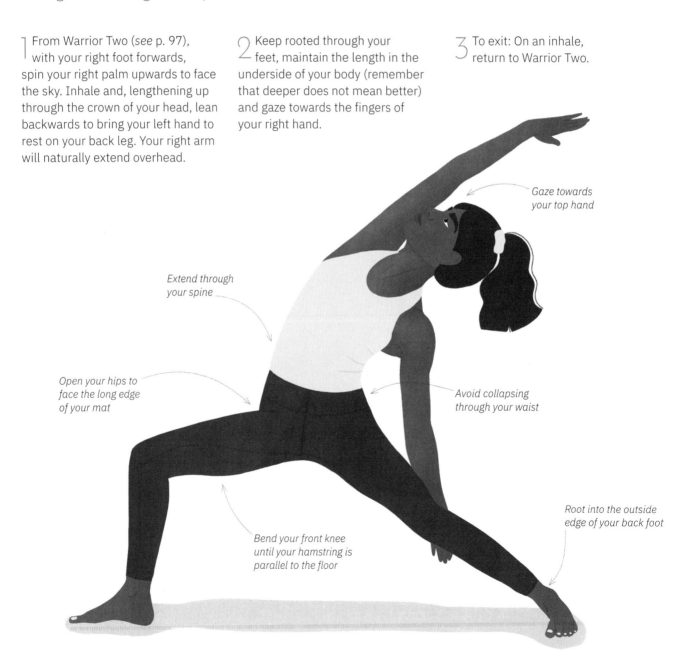

Gaze towards your top hand

Extend through your spine

Open your hips to face the long edge of your mat

Avoid collapsing through your waist

Bend your front knee until your hamstring is parallel to the floor

Root into the outside edge of your back foot

WEEK 3 Abundance
ASTEYA

THE BIG LIE OF MODERN CULTURE is that we don't have enough. That we always need to be striving for more. That we can't afford to rest. That more for you is less for me. That if only we had more time, more money, more success, more possessions, more friends, we would be happy. Our fear of not having enough is rooted in the feeling of not *being* enough. An emptiness. A void. This inner emptiness drives our desire to consume and control and we find ourselves chasing external things, believing they will make us feel whole. But more often than not, when we finally get the promotion or the bigger house or the new relationship, it feels hollow and empty and we are left wanting more.

Practising *asteya* is about recognising our wholeness. Our enoughness. Because when we reconnect with this wholeness, we no longer take more than we need – money, food, attention, other people's time and energy – and we have a natural desire to give where we can.

One sign that we are not living from this state of wholeness is that we hurry through our lives on the rush to nowhere. Although we might not think of it as stealing, by rushing through our lives, we are stealing from ourselves the experience of being fully alive in each moment. We judge the success of our day on how many things we have ticked off our to-do list without being fully present for any of them. We focus on the measurable instead of the meaningful. We cram our days with so much that there is literally no room for living. Practising *asteya* reminds us not to steal our own happiness from ourselves. We won't find that deep, inner joy when we get to the end of our to-do list, but in the ordinary moments of daily life when we are fully present with ourselves and one another in the most loving and caring way.

At the deepest level, the practice of *asteya* asks us to release the desire to have or steal anything that does not belong to us and inspires us to look at all the subtle ways we may be stealing from ourselves, each other and the natural world. Feelings of envy or jealousy are a message that we are living from a place of emptiness instead of wholeness. Even by saying, 'I wish I had that car', 'I wish I had her body', 'I wish I were that famous', we have stolen. By comparing what we have and how we look to others, we are stealing our own happiness. As former US President Teddy Roosevelt famously said, 'Comparison is the thief of joy.'

As we practise living with the attitude of *asteya* – non-stealing, gratitude, generosity, abundance, enoughness – in our daily lives, we begin to see that everything we need is within us. We recognise how staying within our comfort zone is stealing our potential from ourselves and our gifts from the world and so we begin to move beyond it. Instead of looking outside of ourselves for happiness, attention or approval, we begin to look within; to listen to our inner self and experience the deep, inner joy that we can never find in external things.

Asteya is a delicate practice of taking what we need so that we can reach our full potential and be of service to one another and the world without taking more than is necessary. And, like any new skill, we must practise. As often as we can. Daily, if possible. Until it becomes our way of being. Our first task is simply to be aware of those moments when we act from a place of scarcity or lack and to remind ourselves there is enough and we are enough.

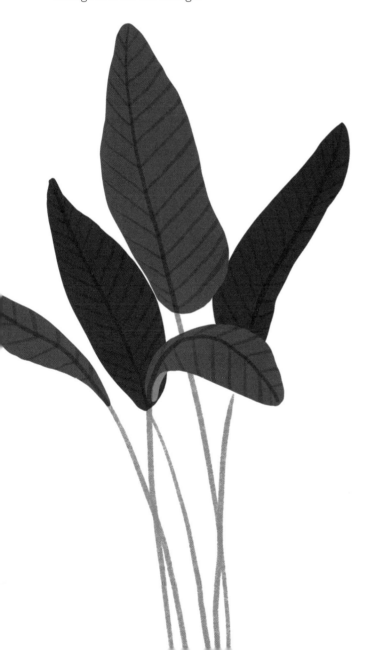

Mindful Living Practice

Journal prompts

Being aware of the ways in which we live from a place of scarcity instead of wholeness can help us see where we may be stealing – time, money, potential, talent, opportunity – from ourselves and others. As our awareness grows, we can begin to create daily practices, rooted in the recognition of our wholeness, that cultivate gratitude for what we have and generosity with what we can share. Journalling on the questions below can help you create a practice of *asteya* that is personal to you.

> *In what ways am I trying to fill an internal void with external things?*
>
> *Who do I regularly compare myself to?*
>
> *What gifts am I hiding from the world?*
>
> *How can I practise generosity in my daily life – with myself and others?*

For example, you might realise that you regularly steal your friends' time in order to avoid being on your own. Practising *asteya* would mean learning to feel at peace in solitude so that the time you spend with your friends is rooted in connection instead of distraction. Or you might discover that by always looking for the next big thing – holiday, wedding, new car – you are stealing the simple joys of daily life from yourself. Sometimes the most generous thing we can do is give ourselves the gift of being fully present in our lives.

Aspiration inspiration

Use the ideas below as inspiration to create your own aspirations that will invite you into a more abundant, generous way of being in the world, grounded in the wisdom that you are enough and you have enough.

> *'May I know I am whole.'*
>
> *'May I see that I am enough just the way I am.'*
>
> *'May I trust that everything I need is within me.'*

True needs and false needs

Much of the things we think we need are false needs, learned needs – things society says we need as symbols of our worthiness. For example, the diet industry tries to convince us that we *need* to have a flat stomach so we buy overpriced and ineffective weight-loss teas. The entertainment industry tries to make us believe that we *need* to be constantly stimulated so we pay to watch their movies. And social media tries to persuade us that we *need* fame and followers so we spend more time and money online. But, by chasing these false needs, what are we stealing from ourselves? Time with loved ones? Discovery of our true purpose? Intimate connection? Sharing our gifts? Basic self-care such as sleep, fresh air and exercise?

This week, take some time to identify your true needs and your false needs. This can often take a little while – or a whole lifetime – to untangle. As you begin to recognise the difference, begin practising *asteya* by letting go of the pursuit of false needs that are stealing energy from the things in your life that are truly meaningful and sacred. Acknowledge where you may have been stealing from others – time, attention, ideas – in order to meet these false needs. And notice what happens to your desire for these false needs once your true needs – the ones that will lead to an inner fullness, fulfilment and wholeness – are met.

We get to define what is a true need and false need for us in each moment, but I have found that many people share the same ideas. The lists below are common examples my clients have come up with over the last few years.

True needs: acceptance, autonomy, belonging, challenge, community, connection, creativity, intimacy, food, love, meaning, nature, physical activity, play, purpose, safety, shelter, sleep, sunlight, understanding, water.

False needs: admiration, alcohol, excess wealth, career success, cigarettes, comfort, commercialised entertainment, constant progress, convenience, culturally beautiful body, exotic holidays, fame, fashionable clothes, fast food, followers, movies, power, six-pack, social media, social status.

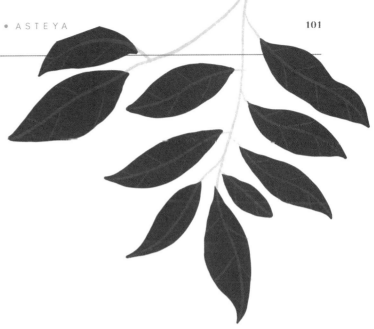

Meditation

Loving Awareness Meditation

Without realising it, we steal love from ourselves many times a day through our self-judgement and harsh self-criticism. We often find ourselves doing this in meditation too: getting frustrated that our mind has wandered and beating ourselves up because we are struggling to pay attention to our breath. This is why the awareness with which we practise has to be a loving awareness. A judgement-free awareness. An unconditionally accepting awareness.

This week, focus on your breath without counting. Do this with a loving awareness so that if thoughts and worries and stories do begin to fill your mind, you can hold them tenderly, with the gentleness you would hold a newborn baby. Instead of fighting them, simply notice that your mind has wandered and bring your awareness – lovingly, tenderly, compassionately, back to your breath. Aim to practise for five to ten minutes; or if you feel like it, take your practice up to 15 or even 20 minutes and be open to whatever arises.

It's helpful to remember that we cannot dwell on the past or worry about the future while focusing on our breath. By practising breath awareness, we are practising awareness of the present moment. We are going nowhere other than right here, returning again and again to the ever-changing, ever-present now.

Asanas: Hip Openers and Hamstrings

ABOUT 25 MINUTES

This week, begin to introduce a short series of hip openers and hamstring stretches into your practice. Use your time on the mat as an opportunity to explore *asteya;* to be fully present in each pose rather than stuck in your head thinking what you should look like in it. When we are constantly striving for more in our practice – which usually comes from a place of not feeling good enough – we rob ourselves of being able to be fully present in our body in each moment. And, if we constantly push too hard and force our body into positions it's simply not ready for, we risk stealing a sustainable, lifelong practice from ourselves owing to injury.

1 **Opening Sequence**
(*p. 58*)

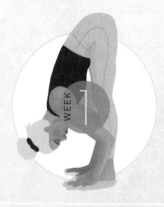

2 Repeat **WEEK 1:**
Standing Forward Bends
(*pp. 86–7*)

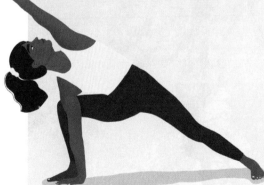

5 **Extended Side Angle Pose,**
5 breaths then transition to
next pose

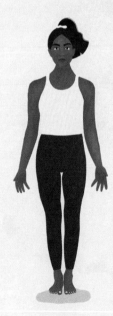

6 **Mountain Pose**
(*p. 64*), 5 breaths

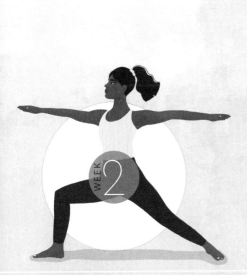

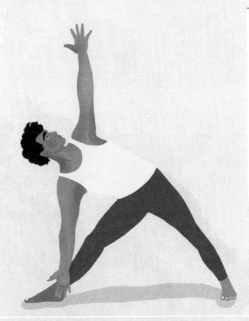

'Transition to next pose' means to move from one pose to the next in a mini-sequence before repeating the same mini-sequence on the left side.

3 Repeat **WEEK 2: Leg-strengthening Poses** (*pp. 94–5*)

4 **Triangle Pose,** 5 breaths then transition to next pose

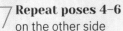

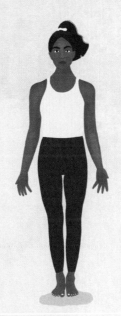

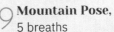

7 **Repeat poses 4–6** on the other side

8 **Pyramid Pose,** 5 breaths each side

9 **Mountain Pose,** 5 breaths

10 **Closing Sequence** (*p. 75*)

Triangle Pose
UTTHITA TRIKONASANA

Remember that deeper isn't always better, so instead of striving for depth in this pose, find a balance between alignment and aliveness.

1 From Mountain Pose (*see* p. 64) step your left foot back roughly one leg-length. Turn your back foot in by about 45 degrees and open your hips to face the long edge of your mat.

2 Ground downwards through both feet and spread your arms out wide in line with your shoulders (this is called Standing Triangle). On an exhalation reach over your front foot and tilt sideways to bring your right hand downwards to rest in front of your knee, shin or ankle. Avoid leaning your weight into your front leg and instead maintain stability through your core.

3 Align your left arm so it is reaching straight up towards the sky and gaze towards your left fingers. Work with your breath, lengthening from your tailbone to crown with each inhalation, and, as you exhale, draw your shoulder blades towards your midline and rotate your chest open towards the sky.

4 To exit: On an inhale, lift your chest back to Standing Triangle.

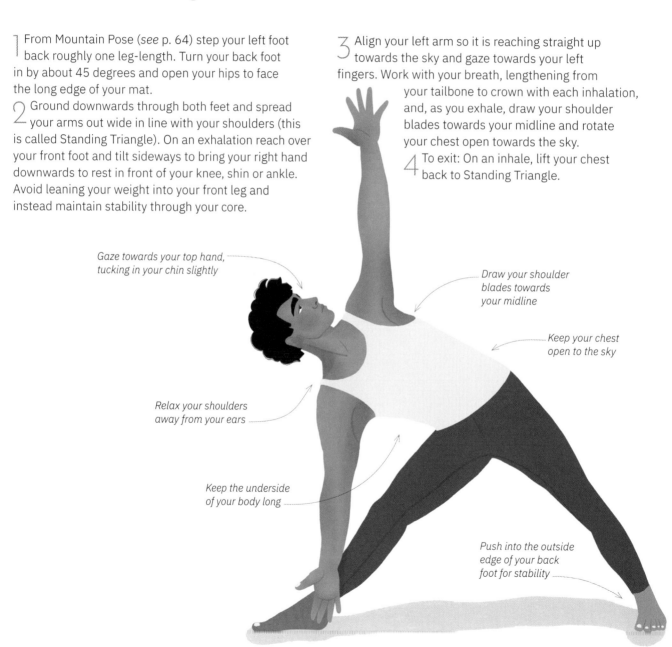

Gaze towards your top hand, tucking in your chin slightly

Draw your shoulder blades towards your midline

Keep your chest open to the sky

Relax your shoulders away from your ears

Keep the underside of your body long

Push into the outside edge of your back foot for stability

Extended Side Angle Pose

UTTHITA PARSVAKONASANA

This pose requires both strength and flexibility. Feel free to place a block on the inside of your front foot if you can't reach the floor.

1 From Standing Triangle (*see opposite*), on an exhalation, bend your front leg and lean forwards to either rest your right forearm on your right thigh (palm facing upwards) or bring your palm to the floor on the inside of your front foot. You can place a block here to give you extra support, if you need it.

2 Shoot your left arm overhead, palm facing downwards, to create a diagonal line of energy from the heel of your left foot through to your left fingertips. Gaze up towards your left hand.

3 Ground downwards through both feet and with each exhalation, see if you can create more openness, rotating upwards from your core.

4 To exit: Push your front foot firmly into the floor and lift your chest as you straighten your front leg back to Standing Triangle.

Once you feel strong in the extended variations, to explore a bind, drop your left arm behind your back and thread your right arm under your right thigh. Clasp your hands and rotate your chest open to look over your left shoulder.

BOUND VARIATION

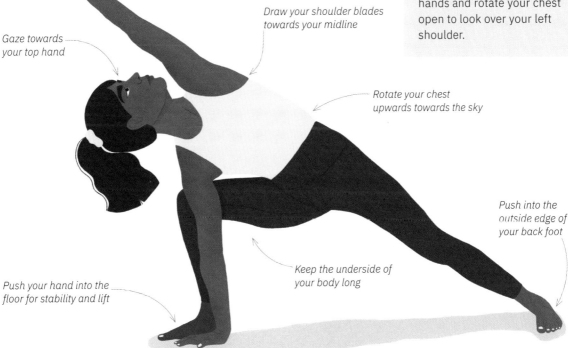

Gaze towards your top hand

Draw your shoulder blades towards your midline

Rotate your chest upwards towards the sky

Push your hand into the floor for stability and lift

Keep the underside of your body long

Push into the outside edge of your back foot

Pyramid Pose

PARSVOTTANASANA

This pose offers a powerful stretch to the hamstrings as well as cultivating focus, calmness and balance.

1 Start in Mountain Pose (*see* p. 64) and step your left leg back, turning your left toes out slightly while keeping your hips facing forwards.

2 Bring your hands to your hips, extending through your spine on an inhalation and as you exhale, fold forwards, placing your hands either side of your front foot (or on blocks if you can't reach the floor).

3 Realign your hips if they have started to spiral open by drawing the thigh bone of your right leg up and into your hip socket and gaze towards the tip of your nose.

4 Work with your breath, finding a subtle extension in your spine as you inhale and drawing deeper into the forward bend as you exhale.

5 To exit: As you inhale, lengthen your spine until it is parallel with the floor. Exhale and bring your hands to your hips and, as you inhale, lift your chest, bending your front knee if you need to. Step your feet together in Mountain Pose before repeating on the other side.

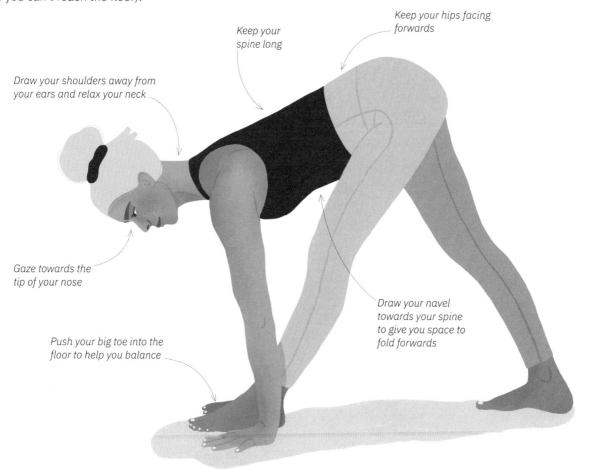

Keep your hips facing forwards

Keep your spine long

Draw your shoulders away from your ears and relax your neck

Gaze towards the tip of your nose

Draw your navel towards your spine to give you space to fold forwards

Push your big toe into the floor to help you balance

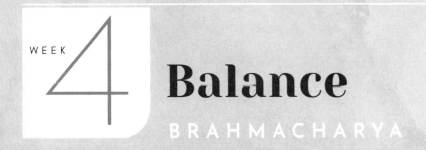

WEEK

4

Balance

BRAHMACHARYA

WE LIVE IN A WORLD OF EXTREMES. Instead of eating a few more vegetables, we go on extreme juice fasts. Instead of enjoying a 20-minute walk around the block, we start training for an ultramarathon. Instead of spending five minutes on social media catching up with our friends, we waste an entire evening scrolling mindlessly through our phones. Instead of eating one cookie, we eat the whole packet.

Over time, doing anything in excess – eating, exercise, sex, dieting, work – drains our energy and pushes us out of balance. And, any contentment we do experience from overeating that extra-large pizza or buying that pair of shoes we couldn't really afford is fleeting, soon to be replaced with guilt for our overindulgence or a desire for more.

The practice of *brahmacharya* asks us to walk the middle path. To find balance instead of ping-ponging from deprivation to overindulgence. It asks us to regulate (not repress) our senses so that we can fully and consciously enjoy all kinds of sensual pleasures – ice cream on a hot summer's day, physical intimacy with someone we love deeply, freshly made coffee at our favourite café – without letting our cravings overpower us. Because, when we are taken over by craving, we move through the world in a kind of trance. We become blind to the simple pleasures of everyday life – the smile from a stranger, the smell of freshly cut grass, the flower growing through the crack in the pavement – because all we can focus on is whatever it is that we think will satisfy our desire. Being able to observe our cravings without acting them out gives us freedom. Rather than being ruled by our desires, we get to *choose* how we live.

Our task, as we begin to practise *brahmacharya*, is to become aware of where we regularly overindulge or deprive ourselves and understand why we do this and how it serves us: to distract, to numb, to suppress. Only then can we begin taming our senses instead of letting them control us.

The literal translation of *brahmacharya* is 'walking in the presence of the divine'. Practically, this means replacing superficial pleasures – those experiences that are immediately rewarding but short-lived such as drinking, smoking and fast food – with divine ones that fill us with aliveness. Imagine the difference between bingeing on ice cream and a moment of deep intimacy and connection with someone you love. Or compare an evening scrolling robotically through your phone to an evening at a salsa class, moving your body in a way that fills you with awe, passion and joy.

Rather than denying ourselves pleasure – which is how *brahmacharya* is sometimes interpreted – we are actually gifting ourselves the deepest, biggest, purest pleasure possible. As we practise *brahmacharya*, what we often find is that we no longer want the superficial pleasures we once craved. We discover that gorging on cookies doesn't bring us any pleasure at all, binge drinking isn't enjoyable, smoking doesn't taste good, over-exercising doesn't feel good and binge watching television isn't really that entertaining after all. And, because we realise these temporary pleasures aren't that pleasurable, we can give them up without a fight.

Through the practice of *brahmacharya* we begin to realise how good it feels to live a life of balance, to take the middle path. By connecting with the part of ourselves that is divine – our deeper and vastly more authentic Self – we begin to see that the superficial pleasures we are giving up are not nearly as good as the things we will discover through our yoga practice: an unshakeable peace, an inner fullness, a deep, spiritual joy.

Mindful Living Practice

Journal prompts

In a world overwhelmed by marketing and subtle messages encouraging us to zigzag from one extreme to the next (I once saw an advert for a triple cheese burger placed next to one for a weight-loss group), it takes conscious self-reflection for us to become mindful of the ways in which we stray from the middle path. Use the questions below to help you become aware of situations and habits where you tend to take things to the extreme. This could be related to food, caffeine, alcohol, work, relationships, shopping, or anything that knocks you off balance and disturbs your peace of mind.

Where do I take things to the extreme through overindulgence?

Where do I take things to the extreme through deprivation?

How can I practise walking the middle path in daily life?

For example, as you reflect, you might realise you are depriving yourself of sleep and drinking far too much coffee, leaving you feeling jittery and exhausted at the same time. Walking the middle path could mean introducing a bedtime routine and sticking to decaffeinated coffee and herbal teas.

Aspiration inspiration

Sometimes we can get addicted to extremes – such as the temporary high of over-exercising and the superficial comfort of scrolling through Instagram – so it's helpful to have an aspiration to remind us of how good it feels when we are living a life of balance. Use the ideas below as inspiration to create your own.

'May I be awake enough to notice when I am taking things to extremes.'

'May I choose deep, spiritual joy over superficial pleasures.'

'May I walk the middle path.'

Mindful indulgence

Yoga is not an ascetic way of life. It does not ask us to avoid pleasure, give up all our belongings and live in a cave in the hope of achieving some kind of non-existent spiritual perfection. In fact, yoga actively encourages us to not only avoid self-indulgence but also avoid self-denial. Rather than depriving yourself of sensual pleasures – by banning chocolate or coffee or sex – this week, allow yourself to be fully present when you are indulging in these experiences.

Choose a food that you would normally deprive yourself of or overindulge in (and then feel guilty about) and practise eating it mindfully. For example, instead of passing on dessert, have a slice of that New York cheesecake your friend made you and enjoy it fully. Eat it slowly. Rest in between mouthfuls. Notice the textures and flavours – the buttery biscuit base, the creamy vanilla filling, the sweet, fruity coulis. Keep checking in with yourself to see whether you want another bite or if it's starting to get a bit sickly and eating more would leave you feeling over-full and bloated. Let your intuition guide you as to when you're straying from the middle path – by over-eating or over-dieting – and mindfully bring yourself back by practising *brahmacharya* and treating your body as sacred.

Breathwork – *pranayama*

Our breath is an ever-present tool we can use to quieten our nervous system and release our cravings for excess. This week, begin to introduce Three-part Breath (*see* p. 112) – traditionally known as *deergha swasam* – to your practice. Most people find it helpful to practise this for five to ten minutes to experience the full benefits. You could do this before or after your *asana* practice, at another set time during the day (like first thing in the morning) or more spontaneously when you notice a craving arise.

Three-part Breath trains us to breathe using our diaphragm – the large muscle that separates the chest and abdominal cavities – instead of relying on the accessory muscles of our chest and neck. This helps to relieve tension, increase our supply of oxygen and calm our nervous system.

Some people find it incredibly helpful to use Three-part Breath at times when they are tempted to overindulge. Simply notice when the craving arises and give yourself full permission to overindulge but only after you have practised five to ten minutes of three-part breathing. After a few minutes of deep, diaphragmatic breathing, many people find their cravings become much more manageable. For detailed instructions on how to practise Three-part Breath, *see* page 112.

Meditation

Anapana - mindfulness of breath

Our meditation practice gives us the opportunity to see when we are off balance. You might notice that your mind is whizzing and whirling at a hundred miles an hour when you've had too much coffee. Or that you can't think about anything but chocolate-chip cookies since you started that extreme low-carb diet. Or that your breath is shallow and sharp since you took on that extra project at work.

As you become more established in your practice, you might also begin to notice physical sensations – heat, cold, heaviness, lightness, itching, throbbing, tingling, contraction, expansion, pleasure, pain, vibration – and how these sensations change depending on your diet, environment, stress levels and whatever thoughts, worries and memories are occurring in the present moment. Perhaps, each time you sit, it feels like you are carrying the weight of the world on your shoulders. Or your skin starts itching. Or there is a pain in your chest that feels like your heart is breaking. Meditation is deeply somatic; fully grounded in the body and the physical sensations that arise. By observing these sensations, we can begin to explore ourselves. We begin to understand, in a truly experiential way, how everything is impermanent; how even the most painful or uncomfortable of sensations will arise and pass away.

This week, introduce *anapana* meditation to your practice. This is a beautifully, simple practice that helps to calm and concentrate the mind and, by focusing on the subtle sensations of the breath, will help you to become more embodied, more present and more aware of when you have fallen out of balance.

Find your seated meditation position, close your eyes and breathe naturally and mindfully. Become aware of the sensation of the breath around the nostrils and the upper lip and focus your attention here. Observe any sensations that occur here. Don't try and find anything extraordinary, simply notice the ordinary physical sensations that arise as you breathe – the coolness of the breath as it enters the nostrils, the heat on your upper lip as you exhale, a subtle tickling at the edge of your nostrils, tingling on the tip of your nose. With a very gentle, loving awareness, and not too much effort, watch these sensations like you are watching a sunset – no judgement, no expectations, no force. And if you catch your mind trying to escape in to the past or future, simply notice that it has wandered and bring your awareness back to the sensation of your breath.

Practise for anything from five to 20 minutes a day this week, noticing how your time in meditation is an invitation for your body to begin showing you things. That, as you stop thinking obsessively, you can begin listening – to your breath, to your body, to the quiet call of your heart.

Asanas: Revolved Standing Poses

ALLOW 25-30 MINUTES

Our physical practice offers us the opportunity to explore the middle path in an embodied way. This week, we introduce three new poses, each requiring a balance between hard work and surrender in order to find stability and balance. As you practise, ask yourself, 'What would I do if I had to hold this pose for 10 minutes? Where would I strengthen? Where would I relax?' By imagining that we have to hold the pose for much longer, we become aware of where we are holding excess tension or trying too hard so that we can release any extreme force and discover a sense of effortless effort in each pose.

1 **Opening Sequence** (*see p. 58*)

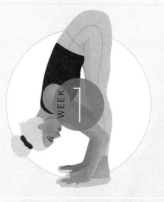

2 Repeat **WEEK 1: Standing Forward Bends** (*see pp. 86–7*)

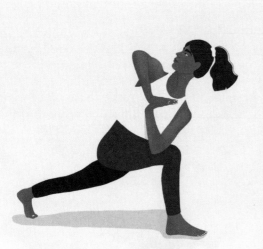

6 **Revolved Side Angle Pose** (*see p. 114*), 5 breaths then transition to next pose

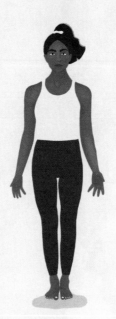

7 **Mountain Pose** (*see p. 64*), 5 breaths

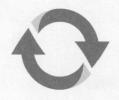

8 **Repeat poses 5–7** on other side

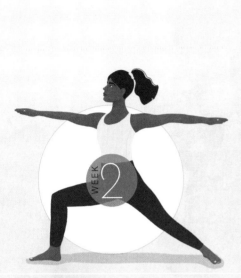

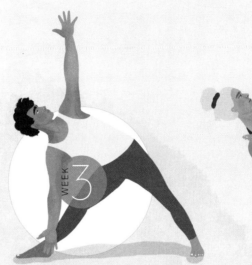

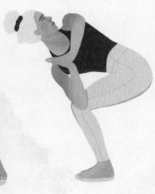

3 Repeat **WEEK 2:**
Leg-strengthening Poses
(*see pp. 94–5*)

4 Repeat **WEEK 3:**
Hip Openers and Hamstring
Stretches (*see pp. 102–3*)

5 **Revolved Chair**
Twist over right leg (*see p. 113*),
five breaths then transition to
next pose by stepping left leg
back while keeping left elbow
squeezed into right leg

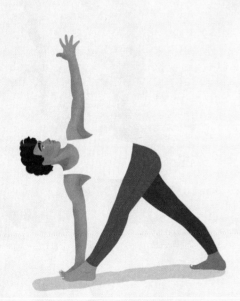

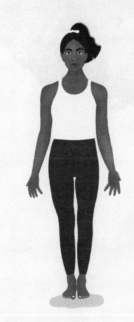

9 **Revolved Triangle Pose**
(*see p. 115*), 5 breaths then
repeat on other side

10 **Mountain Pose,**
5 breaths

11 **Closing Sequence**
(*see p. 75*)

Three-part Breath

DEERGHA SWASAM

This is a calming, grounding breathing exercise that teaches us how to breathe fully and deeply using our diaphragm. Practise this technique lying down before exploring it seated.

1 Either lying on your back or in a seated position, place your hands on your collarbones so that you can feel the movement of your breath.

2 Breathing through your nose, breathe into your belly, feeling it rise like a balloon, and as you exhale, let your navel fall back towards your spine. Take five breaths like this.

3 Now, as you inhale, breathe into your belly and, once the belly is full, expand the ribcage. As you exhale, let your breath release from the ribcage first and then the belly. Take five breaths like this.

4 This time, as you inhale, first feel your belly expand, then your ribcage, and then fill your upper chest, expanding the areas around your collarbones. Exhale in reverse – from your upper chest, then from your ribcage, and then from your belly. Take ten to 15 breaths here, focusing on breathing smoothly and seamlessly.

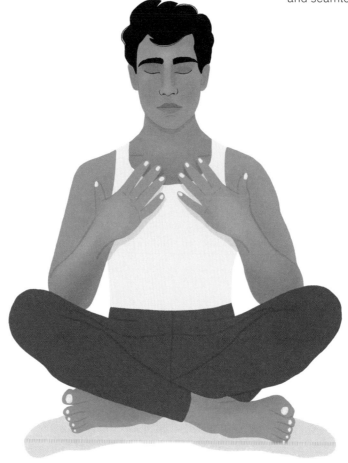

Revolved Chair

PARIVRTTA UTKATASANA

This is a powerful pose, increasing mobility in the spine and providing a sense of both grounding and openness.

1 From Chair Pose (*see* p. 73) bring your palms to your heart and, as you exhale, bring your left elbow to the outside of your right thigh, twisting from your waist and maintaining length in your spine.

2 Make sure your knees are in alignment, squeezing your inner thighs towards each other for stability, and on each exhale, twist a little deeper into the pose, pushing your palms together and drawing your elbows apart. Gaze over your right shoulder.

3 To exit: Rotate back to centre before repeating on the other side.

In this sequence, transition from Revolved Chair to Revolved Side Angle Pose (*see* p. 114) by maintaining the twist and stepping your left leg back.

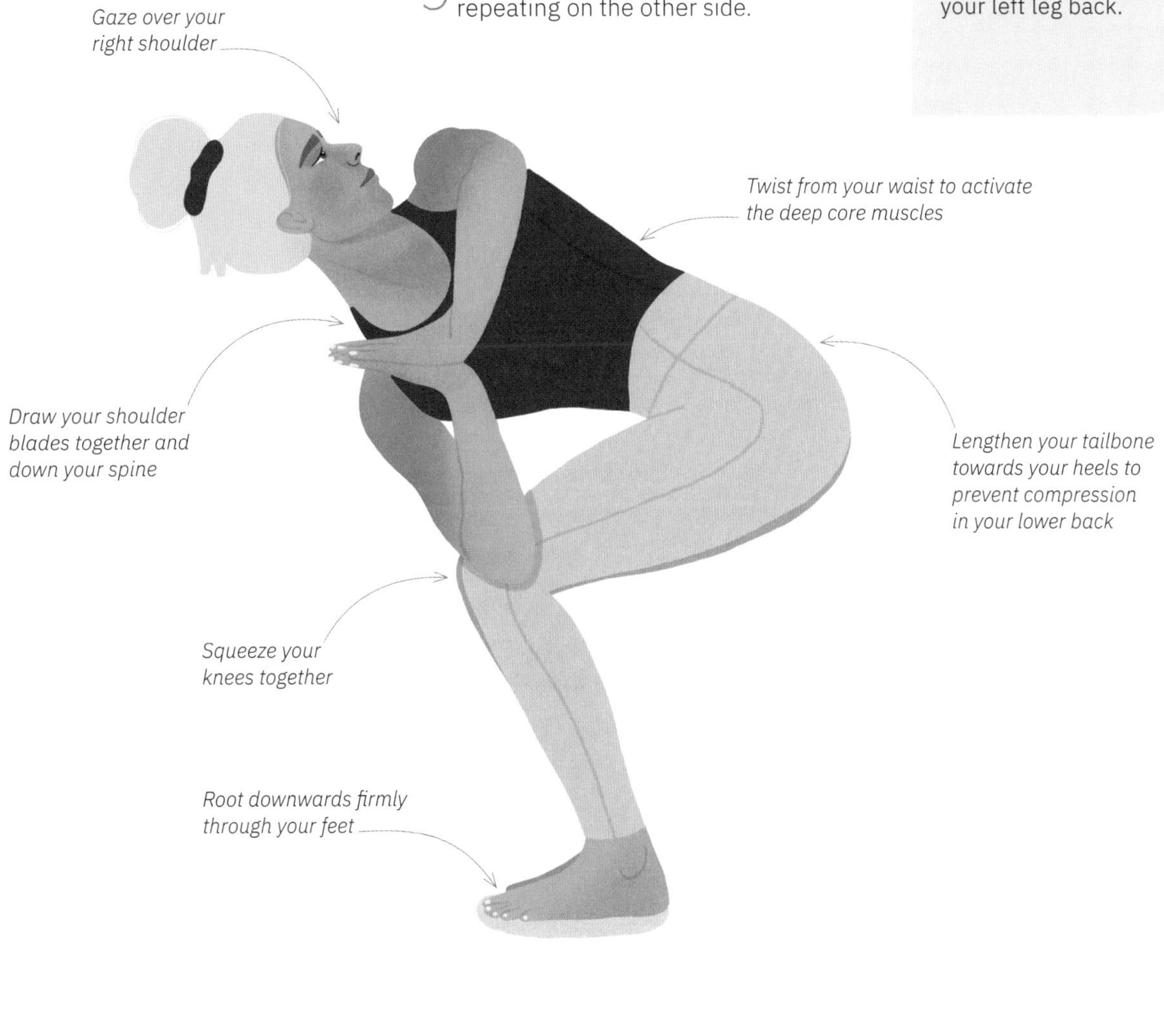

TRANSITION NOTE

Gaze over your right shoulder

Twist from your waist to activate the deep core muscles

Draw your shoulder blades together and down your spine

Lengthen your tailbone towards your heels to prevent compression in your lower back

Squeeze your knees together

Root downwards firmly through your feet

Revolved Side Angle Pose

PARIVRTTA PARSVAKONASANA

Instead of striving for the deepest twist possible, focus on creating stability and then fully breathing into the pose.

1 From Revolved Chair (*see* p. 114), twisting to your right and squeezing your left elbow into the outside of your right thigh, mindfully step your left leg about one leg-length backwards and then refine your position.

2 Make sure your right elbow is pointing towards the sky and rotate to bring your breastbone up to meet your thumbs. Gaze over your right shoulder.

3 Work with your breath to twist deeper into the pose on each exhalation while maintaining a sense of lift. If this is difficult, drop your back knee to the ground.

4 To exit: Either step forward to Revolved Chair or release the twist, bring your hands to the floor either side of your front foot ,and step back to Downward Dog (*see* p. 72) or forward to Mountain Pose (*see* p.64).

> **PRACTICE TIP**
>
> **If you are creating** your own sequence, you can also enter the pose from Warrior One (*see* p. 74) by bringing your hands to your heart and lengthening through your spine to create space around your waist. On an exhalation, root down firmly through your back foot and twist through your core to bring your left elbow to the outside of your right thigh.

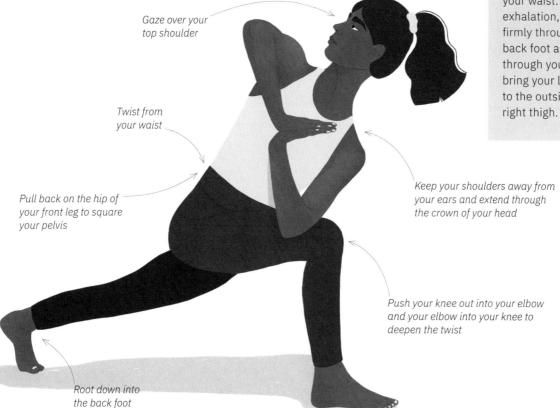

Gaze over your top shoulder

Twist from your waist

Pull back on the hip of your front leg to square your pelvis

Keep your shoulders away from your ears and extend through the crown of your head

Push your knee out into your elbow and your elbow into your knee to deepen the twist

Root down into the back foot

Revolved Triangle Pose

PARIVRTTA TRIKONASANA

This is a challenging pose that combines a forward bend, a balance and a twist.
Use props to help you find your natural alignment if you need to.

1 Begin in Mountain Pose (*see* p. 64) and step
your left foot back, turning the toes out slightly
while keeping your hips facing forwards. Place
your right hand on your hip and reach your left
arm out in front of you.

2 Activate your legs for stability and as you
exhale, reach forwards and downwards
with your left arm, placing your left hand either on
the inside or outside of your right foot. You can use
a block here if reaching the ground is challenging.

3 Twist from your waist and extend your right arm
towards the sky, gazing up to your right fingers.

4 Keep lengthening from your tailbone through the
crown of your head, grounding firmly through both
feet, and gently deepen the twist as you exhale by
rotating your torso upwards towards the sky.

5 To exit: Lower your right hand to the floor and slowly
lift your chest back up to standing, stepping your feet
together to return to Mountain Pose before repeating
on the other side.

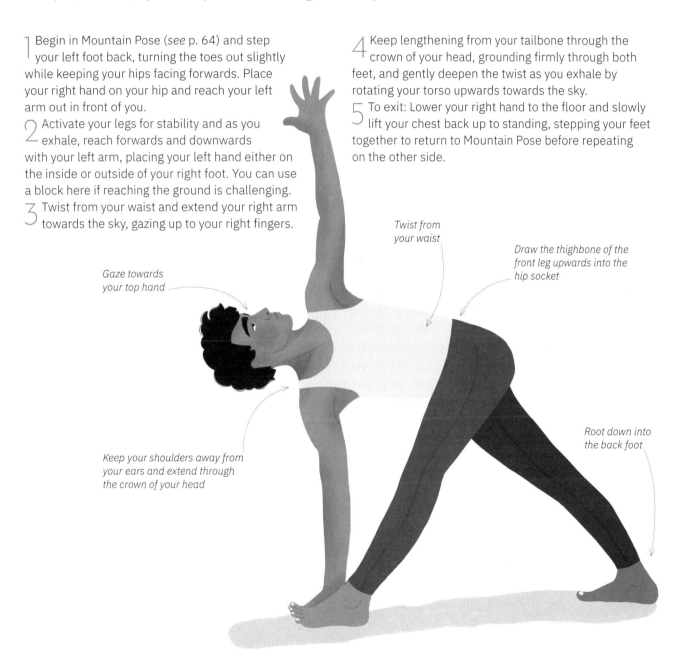

*Twist from
your waist*

*Draw the thighbone of the
front leg upwards into the
hip socket*

*Gaze towards
your top hand*

*Keep your shoulders away from
your ears and extend through
the crown of your head*

*Root down into
the back foot*

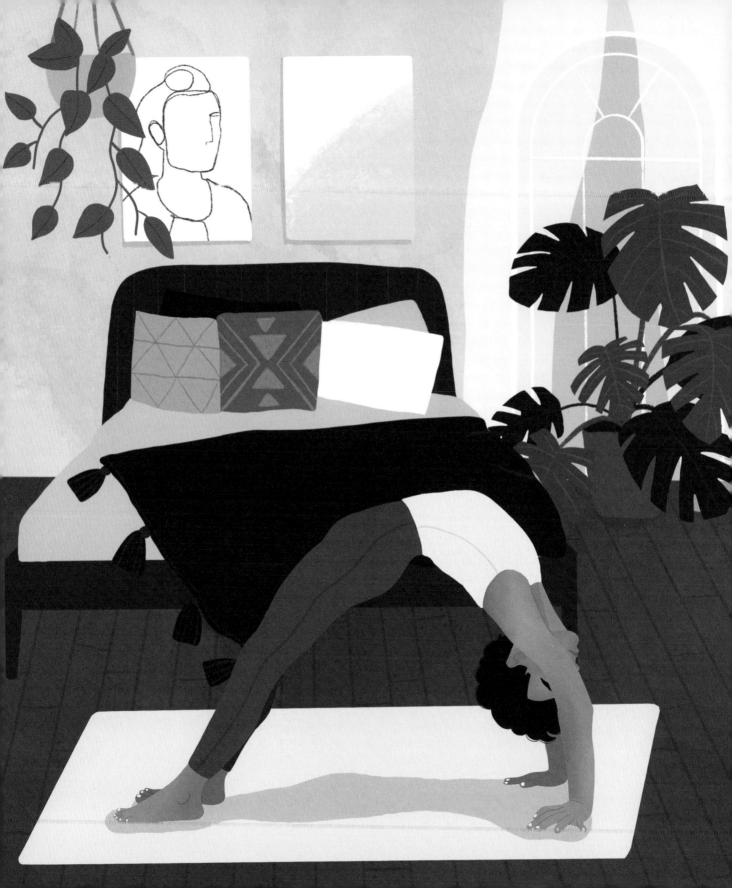

5 Non-attachment

APARIGRAHA

APARIGRAHA IS LARGELY A PRACTICE IN LETTING GO. Of releasing what no longer serves us. Of holding ourselves a little more lightly so we can create space for who we can become. It asks us to stop clinging to people, possessions and beliefs, to be aware instead of attached, to accept the impermanence of everything. Ultimately, the practice of *aparigraha* is about freedom. The freedom to choose instead of being enslaved to destructive habits. The freedom to love another without possessing or controlling them. The freedom to give ourselves fully to each moment without attachment to an outcome or a fantasy of how things 'should' be.

Most of us struggle with non-attachment – with letting go of the things we have outgrown and trusting that everything will be okay when we do – but we have to ask ourselves whether our possessiveness is serving us. How is our habit of clinging – to a relationship, a job, an identity – causing us to suffer? How would it feel to stop grasping for more? How much suffering would we free ourselves from if we were to let go of our attachment to things that are beyond our control, such as other people's behaviour, the shape of our body, the price of petrol, the past, the weather, the traffic.

Without conscious practice, the normal state of the human mind is one of attachment that leads to suffering because, at the end of the day, we can't hold onto anything. All things come and go, arise and pass away. *Aparigraha* invites us to experience the world in a way that allows, accepts and embraces change. And, because we accept the impermanence of everything, we can love it fully while it is here and, when the time comes, we can peacefully and gracefully let it go.

A Buddhist story known as *The Broken Teacup* teaches the power of non-attachment beautifully.

The story goes that the Buddha, when asked by one of his students about how to cultivate greater spiritual freedom by no longer clinging to things, replied: 'Every morning, I drink from my favourite teacup. I enjoy the beauty of the cup and the warmth, aroma and taste of the tea fully. But, in my mind, the teacup is already broken.' The truth is, teacups will break, relationships will end, bodies will change, faces will age, people we love will die, identities will be outgrown and things won't always go to plan. The more attached we are to how things are now or how we think things should be, the more likely we are to suffer.

It's worth highlighting that non-attachment is not the same as detachment. Practising *aparigraha* will not turn us into detached, non-caring flesh robots. In fact, it does the opposite. It allows us to embrace life fully and openly without having a fixed idea of how things should be, to love deeply while letting each other be free, to cherish each joyful moment because we know just how precious and fleeting every moment is.

Practising *aparigraha* teaches us how pointless it is to cling so tightly to things that are so transitory and that, when we do, we become trapped in a too-small life. When we find ourselves hoarding belongings or stubbornly clinging to beliefs, it is a call for us to pay attention to what is going on at a deeper level. What are we afraid of? Not having what we need? Not being loved? Not knowing who we are? Often, when we become disconnected from our true Self, we tend to seize whatever external things we can – people, possessions, identities, beliefs – and hold onto them for dear life. But, when we are deeply connected to our inner world, it's easier to let go of whatever we are attached to because we know on a level deeper than words that nothing outside of us can make us whole.

Mindful Living Practice

Journal prompts

When we look at ourselves deeply, most of us will find that we are attached to lots of things and that these attachments and subtle addictions are causing us to suffer. Many of us believe that if we get the promotion, or if we had enough money, or if the man or woman of our dreams swept us off our feet, we would be happy and all our problems would be solved for ever. However, if we do get these things, we usually discover the happiness they bring is fleeting, we begin to suffer from the fear of losing them, and we start craving something else. Use the questions below to help you reflect on what you are attached to and how you can practise letting go in daily life.

What am I attached to (possessions, people, identities, beliefs)?

How do my attachments imprison me?

How can I practise letting go of my attachments in my daily life?

An example might be: 'I am attached to my identity as a lawyer, my income, and the luxuries it allows me to have in life. But I dread going to work every day, constantly feel exhausted and have no time to exercise or look after my health. These attachments are keeping me imprisoned in a life I don't truly want to live. I can practise non-attachment by looking at other career opportunities that are more in line with my values and by simplifying my life of luxuries that I don't really need so I don't feel pressurised to work so much in order to afford to have them.'

Aspiration inspiration

Use the ideas below to create your own aspirations to open you to the possibility that you can be happy without the things you thought you needed to make you happy.

'May I have the courage to release what no longer serves me.'

'May I love in such a way that the person I love feels free.'

'May I create space in my life for the person I can become.'

Mindful decluttering

Owning nice things and having lots of possessions is not the problem. It is our relationship with these things that can cause us to suffer if we expect to find happiness in buying and possessing them. And, while giving away all our stuff is not going to bring us freedom if our mind is still trapped in a state of attachment and craving, having a mindful declutter can create space in our head as well as our home.

This week, spend five minutes a day decluttering your home. As you go through your wardrobes and bookshelves and kitchen cupboards, hold each item and ask yourself: 'Is this item useful?', 'Is it beautiful?', 'Is it worth the space it is taking up?', 'Does it bring me joy?' If the answer is no to all of these questions, maybe it is time to let it go.

Meditation

Earth Breathing

Oftentimes, we find ourselves clinging to things when we don't feel grounded in our body or on the Earth; when we don't trust ourselves or our intuitions; when we think we need something outside of ourselves to keep us safe and bring us happiness. Earth Breathing is a body-based meditation practice that helps us to root ourselves deeply in our own body and connects us with the Earth

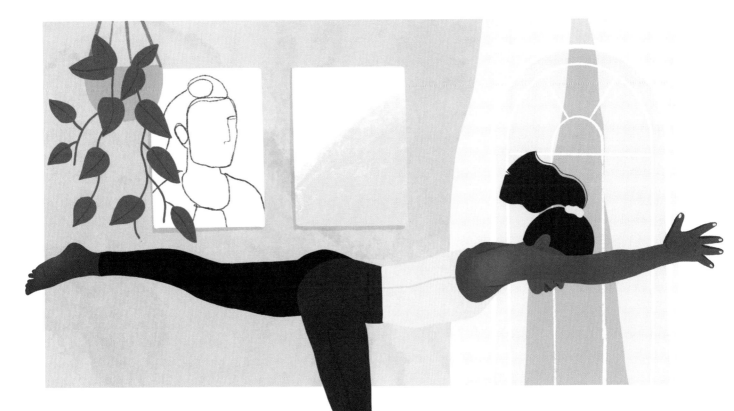

as a source of strength, protection and belonging.

Begin in your seated meditation position, close your eyes and bring your awareness to your perineum – the area between your sitting bones, in between the genitals and anus. Many people find they hold a lot of tension here, so see if you can relax this area, allowing your sitting bones to sink down into your meditation cushion or the ground beneath you. This letting go can sometimes feel quite vulnerable and you may find yourself escaping into thoughts and judgements, which often results in a retightening of the perineum. If this happens, simply come back into your body, tuning in to the tension in your perineum and releasing it.

Next, begin breathing by feeling and visualising yourself breathing up through your perineum from underneath you, and as you exhale, feel your sitting bones relax even more deeply towards the Earth. After a few breaths, begin to drop your awareness about 30cm beneath you into the Earth below, breathing up Earth

energy as you inhale, and relaxing your perineum and descending downwards into the Earth as you exhale. Keep dropping your awareness deeper into the Earth – 60cm, a metre, 2 metres, 3 metres, 30 metres, 300 metres. Breathe upwards from the depths of the Earth and sink deeper into this peaceful, open, safe space as you exhale.

If you find yourself lost in thought, overwhelmed by long-forgotten memories or overcome by intense emotions, let them be there and drop your awareness back into the depth of your body and the depth of the Earth, letting go and relaxing into this unfamiliar universe within.

You can practise this for anywhere between ten minutes to one hour, descending deeper and deeper into the wild mystery of your body and the Earth that holds you. As you come out of this practice, you may want to finish with a couple of minutes of Loving Awareness Meditation (see p. 101), staying connected to the sacredness of this body, this life and this earth.

Asanas: Standing Balances

ALLOW 30-35 MINUTES

We can become so attached to our physical practice – to practising a certain number of times a week or to achieving a certain pose – that we forget the essence of our practice. The new poses this week are standing balances, which offer us the opportunity to bring *aparigraha* to the mat; to release our attachment to the outcome of our practice and, instead, give ourselves completely to it.

1 Opening Sequence
(*see p. 58*)

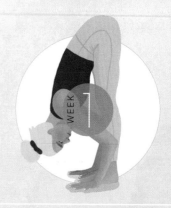

**2 Repeat WEEK 1:
Standing Forward Bends**
(*see pp. 86–7*)

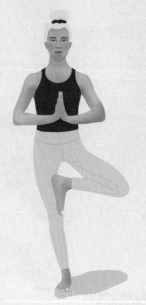

6 Tree Pose
(*see p. 122*),
5 breaths then repeat on other side

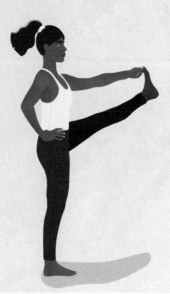

7 Hand to Big Toe Balance A
or **Knee to Chest Balance A**
(*see p. 123*), 5 breaths then transition to next pose

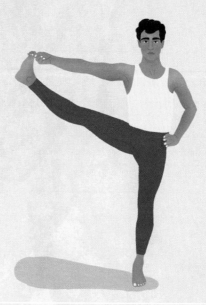

8 Hand to Big Toe Balance B
or **Knee to Chest Balance B**
(*see p. 124*), 5 breaths then transition to next pose.

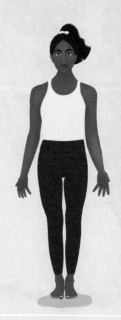

9 Mountain Pose
(*see p. 64*),
5 breaths

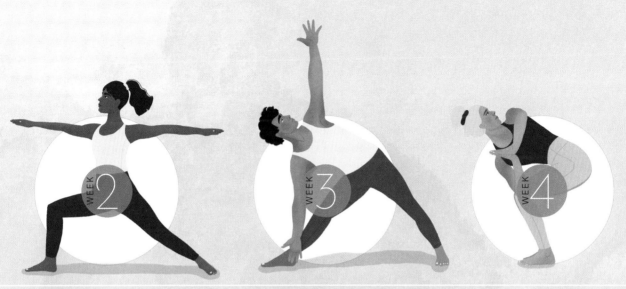

3 Repeat **WEEK 2:**
Leg-strengthening Poses
(*see pp. 94–5*)

4 Repeat **WEEK 3:**
Hip Openers and **Hamstring**
Stretches (*see pp. 102–3*)

5 Repeat **WEEK 4:**
Revolved Standing Poses
(*see pp. 110–11*)

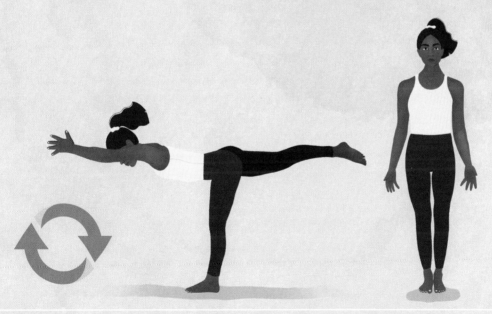

10 **Repeat poses 7–9**
on other side.

11 **Warrior Three**
(*see p. 125*), 5 breaths
then repeat on
other side

12 **Mountain Pose,**
5 breaths

13 **Closing Sequence**
(*see p. 75*)

Tree Pose

VRKSASANA

This is a strong pose that teaches us the importance of staying grounded and rooted in order to find balance

1 Begin in Mountain Pose (*see* p. 64) and shift your weight into your left foot, rooting downwards firmly. Lift your right foot off the floor, bend your right knee and rotate outwards from the hip to place the sole of your foot on your inner calf or inner thigh.

2 Push your left foot firmly into the floor, lengthening your tailbone towards the floor, and lift upwards out of your pelvis.

3 Bring your palms to your heart and gaze straight ahead.

4 To exit: return to Mountain Pose (*see* p.64).

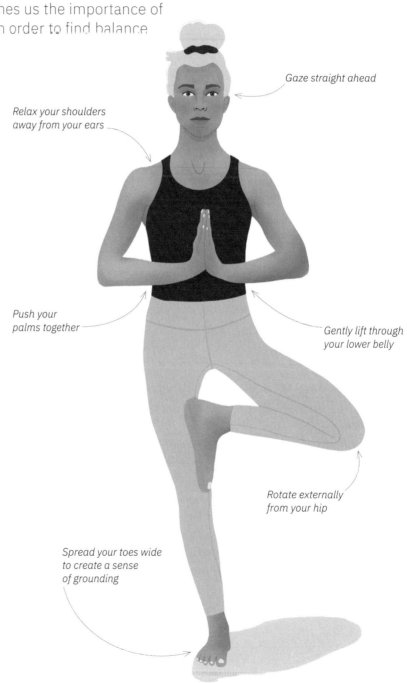

Gaze straight ahead

Relax your shoulders away from your ears

Push your palms together

Gently lift through your lower belly

Rotate externally from your hip

Spread your toes wide to create a sense of grounding

Hand to Big Toe Balance A

UTTHITA HASTA PADUNGUSTHASANA

This pose requires steadiness and openness. Straightening the lifted leg is often challenging to begin with so start off by exploring the bent-knee variation below if you need to.

1 From Mountain Pose (*see* p. 64) shift your weight into your left foot and lift your right leg, bending the knee and drawing your thigh towards your chest. Wrap your hands around your shin and lengthen your spine.

2 Once you feel stable here, walk your hands down your shin towards your foot, either taking hold of the right big toe with your right index and middle fingers or gripping the outside of your foot with your right hand. Bring your left hand to your left hip.

3 On an exhalation, extend your right leg directly out in front of you, drawing your thigh bone back in to your hip socket to keep you centred. Gaze straight ahead or towards your right foot.

4 To exit: Transition straight into Hand to Big Toe Balance B (*see* p.124) by taking your leg out to the side.

Gaze straight ahead or towards your foot

Relax your shoulders away from your ears

Draw your thigh bone back into your hip socket

Extend from your tailbone to your crown

Spread your toes wide to create a sense of grounding

VARIATION

KNEE TO CHEST BALANCE A

TADASANA PAWANMUKTASANA

This is a challenging pose for many people, especially if you have tight hamstrings, so a great alternative is keeping the knee bent and hugging your thigh to your chest by clasping your hands around your shin. Focus on extending from your tailbone to the crown of your head.

Hand to Big Toe Balance B

UTTHITA PARSVASAHITA

1 From Hand to Big Toe Balance A (see p. 123), on an exhalation take your leg out to the side to form a Y-shape. Keep your hips even by dropping the right hip slightly and pushing your left foot firmly into the floor.

2 Gaze to look ahead or over your left shoulder.

3 Come back to Hand to Big Toe Balance A before releasing to Mountain Pose (see p. 64).

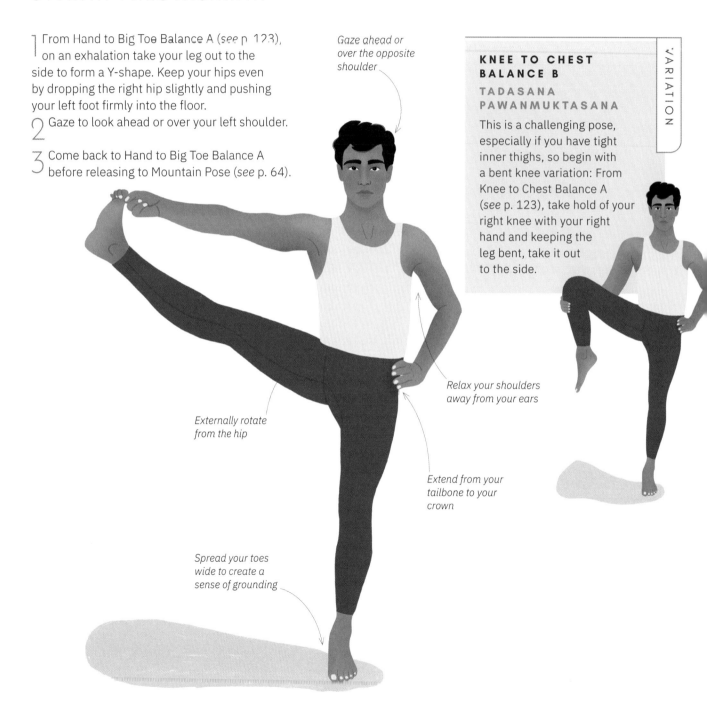

Gaze ahead or over the opposite shoulder

Relax your shoulders away from your ears

Externally rotate from the hip

Extend from your tailbone to your crown

Spread your toes wide to create a sense of grounding

VARIATION

KNEE TO CHEST BALANCE B

TADASANA PAWANMUKTASANA

This is a challenging pose, especially if you have tight inner thighs, so begin with a bent knee variation: From Knee to Chest Balance A (see p. 123), take hold of your right knee with your right hand and keeping the leg bent, take it out to the side.

Warrior Three

VIRABHADRASANA C

This is a challenging pose for most people. Stay balanced by finding a spot on the floor to gaze at.

1. From Mountain Pose (*see* p. 64) bring your hands to your heart in prayer position and shift your weight into your left foot. Tip your upper body forwards at the same time as lifting your right leg up behind you until both your torso and right leg are parallel to the floor. Push your standing foot firmly into the floor and straighten your standing leg.

2. Lengthen your tailbone towards your heels to prevent you dumping into your lower back and either stretch your arms out towards the sides or extend them overhead, shoulder-width apart.

3. Gaze downwards to the floor or to the tip of your nose, spreading your weight evenly between all four corners of your standing foot to help you balance.

4. To exit: Lift your chest as you lower your back leg to return to Mountain Pose before repeating on the other side.

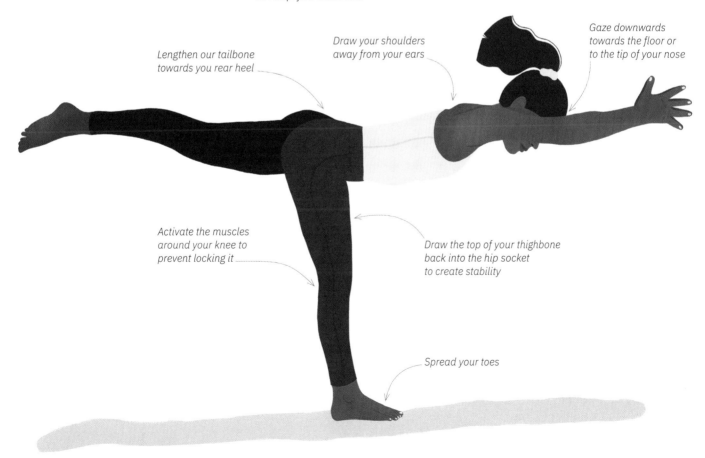

Lengthen our tailbone towards you rear heel

Draw your shoulders away from your ears

Gaze downwards towards the floor or to the tip of your nose

Activate the muscles around your knee to prevent locking it

Draw the top of your thighbone back into the hip socket to create stability

Spread your toes

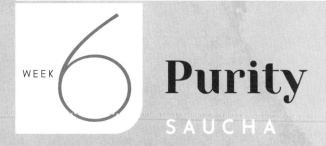

WEEK 6

Purity

SAUCHA

AS WE MOVE FURTHER into our yoga journey, we draw our awareness inwards. Our focus deepens to not only include our relationships with others and external things – non-harm, non-lying, non-stealing, non-excess and non-attachment – but also our relationship with ourselves. It is only by looking at ourselves with this radical honesty that we can begin to see the habits that disturb our inner peace and thinking patterns that enslave us. Once we recognise these destructive habits and limiting beliefs, we can start to do the inner work required to let go of them. And once we let go of them, we will discover that underneath the fragments of self-doubt and shards of unworthiness, we have been whole all along.

Saucha – purity – is the first of the *niyamas*, practices that teach us how to see ourselves more clearly and love ourselves more deeply. It is the paradoxical practice of both purifying ourselves through physical and mental hygiene practices and accepting, welcoming and integrating all that is impure within us – the messy, mysterious, rejected, shame-filled parts that we have banished to the shadows.

We can begin practising *saucha* in a very embodied way by paying attention to our body and how it responds to what we eat and drink. Maybe bread makes you feel sluggish. Or your triple espresso causes a midday energy crash. Or the large glass of wine you've got into the habit of drinking every evening clouds your thinking and leaves you feeling down. As we become more aware of the way in which different food and drink impacts our emotions, shifts our energy and influences our behaviours, we are given the opportunity to nourish ourselves in a way that leads to greater health and wholeness. This isn't about cleansing or detoxing in an attempt to achieve a pure, perfect body. Rather, *saucha* is about realising our body

is a changing, ageing, decaying thing worthy of our deepest care and respect.

There is no judgement in the practice of *saucha*. No food is good or bad. No body is right or wrong. There is simply a blossoming awareness of what takes us away from our natural state of health and wholeness and what unites us with it. Listening to the messages our body is telling us – eating when we are hungry, stopping when we are full, focusing on wholefoods that fill us with a grounded, peaceful energy and staying away from foods that leave us feeling anxious or sluggish – brings with it a beautiful kind of freedom. The freedom from judgement. The freedom to trust our appetite, our intuition and our body. The freedom to experience true health and wholeness and to inspire those around us to do the same. You can find more information on the yoga of eating on page 54.

As well as being mindful of the foods we are eating, the practice of *saucha* asks us to be aware of what we are feeding our mind: the thoughts we think, the television programmes we watch and the media we consume.

Does your favourite crime drama disturb your peace of mind? Does the personal trainer you follow on Instagram leave you feeling unworthy? After reading that celebrity magazine, do you find yourself wanting the designer handbag or the luxury holiday or the latest iPhone? Do you find yourself thinking, 'I'll be happy when...'?

When we begin to pay attention to our thoughts and cravings, we see how much of what we think we want, we have been conditioned to want. And it is this conditioning that stains and distorts our way of seeing the world and causes us to suffer. Much of the practice of *saucha* asks us to untangle what is natural and wholesome within ourselves and what thoughts and behaviours stem from our conditioning so that we can become the purest, most authentic versions of ourselves.

Purity does not mean perfect. It means real. It means raw. It means naked. It means true. It means whole. It means coming home to who we really are beneath everything we have been told we should be. It means reclaiming the outcast fragments of ourselves: the messy, the mysterious, the beautifully imperfect and the vibrantly alive.

Mindful Living Practice

Journal prompts

Sometimes, it isn't until we give ourselves space to reflect that we begin to see the ways in which external things – food, drink, television shows, social media – disturb our peace of mind and distance us from our true Self. Use the questions below to help you explore any habits that might be taking you away from your natural state of health and wholeness and any practices you could begin to implement in your daily life to bring you closer to it.

What foods and drinks leave me feeling sluggish and which leave me feeling energised?

How can I eat in a way that embraces the practice of saucha*?*

What media am I regularly consuming that disturbs my peace of mind?

How can I practise saucha *through the types of television show I watch and media I consume?*

For example, you might realise that following certain people on social media triggers feelings of jealousy and insecurity and the healthiest and most wholesome thing you could do is unfollow them.

Aspiration inspiration

Use the aspirations below to inspire you to create your own around the concept of *saucha*. It's often helpful to repeat them first thing in the morning and last thing at night, as well at any time when you experience cravings for something that will take you away from health and wholeness.

'May I release any habits that take me away from my natural state of health and wholeness.'

'May I welcome all parts of myself.'

'May I stop striving for perfection and come home to who I am.'

Loving the parts that have not known love

Another way to practise *saucha* is to welcome the parts of ourselves untouched by love. The places within us wrapped in shame and unworthiness. The parts we suppress and reject and hide because we believe they are impure, defective, wrong. We cannot cut off parts of ourselves and expect to feel whole. It is only by welcoming these outcast parts of our souls that we can let ourselves be fully seen, fully found, fully loved and fully held.

Make a list of all the things you dislike about yourself; the shadow parts you usually hide from others (and maybe yourself too). Become curious about these parts of yourself. Bring them out into the light. How have they served you? How have they protected you? How can you accept them? How can you transform them? What gifts are hiding within them? As we welcome the discarded parts of ourselves, we begin to become our purest, truest, most authentic Self. Our shame, our unworthiness, our regret, our grief – learning to love it all, that was the gift all along.

Breathwork – *pranayama*

There are many traditional cleansing practices in yoga – known as *kriyas* – and a breathing technique called *kapalabhati* is one of the most beautiful and the most poworful. *Kapalabhati* is translated as 'skull shining breath' because it clears the nasal passages and sinuses and increases oxygenation in the brain, metaphorically making the 'skull shine'!

Kapalabhati is an energising, heating breath so it is best to practise it in the morning, before your yoga practice or if you find yourself feeling sluggish throughout the day. It focuses on the exhalation by making it active and powerful in contrast to the more passive exhalation in Victorious Breath (*see* p.63) or Equal Breathing (*see* p.62).

In essence, *kapalabhati* is a steady repetition of powerful exhalations propelled by forcefully contracting the abdomen, quickly followed by an effortless inhalation as the abdomen is relaxed. If you're new to *kapalabhati*, as you practise you might find it helpful to imagine the kind of forceful exhalation you'd do if a bug flew up one of your nostrils or to visualise blowing out the candles on a birthday cake through your nose. You can find detailed instructions for *kapalabhati* on page 132.

Meditation

Ten-point Meditation

Many of us in the Western world go through our days as a walking head, a brain on a stick. We have become so alienated from our own bodies that we don't know when we are hungry or full, which foods energise us and which leave us bloated and lethargic, when we need movement and when we need rest. Meditation is a gateway back into the body; a tool we can use to reclaim an intimate and loving relationship with our body. A relationship where we can begin to remove our muscular armour; to release the tension in our muscles that have tightened as a way of protecting ourselves from life. A relationship where the body becomes a teacher. One that does not communicate with us through thoughts or language but speaks to us in a direct, naked way through sensations, feelings, intuitions, images, visions and somatic memories.

This week, introduce Ten-point Meditation to your practice. This is an embodied meditation that helps us learn how to come out of our head and into our body; to release tension, awaken sensation and develop a sense of grounding. The ten points we bring our awareness to in this practice are the head, the two shoulder blades, the two elbows, the mid-back, the two buttocks and the two feet, focusing on releasing any tension downwards into the Earth.

Begin in your seated meditation posture, close your eyes and bring your awareness to the crown of your head. Imagine that someone is pouring a soothing, golden oil over your skull that flows downwards, relaxing everything it touches, dissolving any tension, melting any tightness. Relax your forehead, your eye sockets, your cheeks and jaw. Feel this soothing oil flow down the back of your neck, becoming aware of any tension in your shoulder blades and releasing it. Now feel the oil flow down to your elbows and your mid-back. Take a moment to feel the tension here and then release it, letting it dissolve downwards. Move down your spine and feel the soothing oil flood your pelvic area. Explore this region of the body. Notice any tension and then release and relax downwards, feeling the sitting bones sink into the Earth. Feel the soothing, golden oil travel downwards towards your feet, noticing any tension in your thighs, knees and shins and releasing it downwards, like a current of energy flowing into the Earth. Pay attention to the different areas of your feet: the soles, the big toes, the little toes and all the toes in between. One by one, notice the sensations here, feel the tension and let it dissolve, melting downwards. Repeat this process as many times as you need to, beginning at the top of the head and letting the soothing oil flow over and through you. Tension manifests when we are not aware of it, so keep finding places where you're clenching, holding or resisting and relax them, constantly releasing downwards through your buttocks, your feet, anywhere that is touching the ground, into the Earth.

As you practise you may notice how exhausting it is to hold on to tension. Give yourself permission to let go. Releasing. Relaxing. Melting. Dissolving. Letting the Earth hold you. Getting to know yourself deeply. Reconnecting with your body so you can begin to experience the world with your whole being in a beautifully raw and naked way.

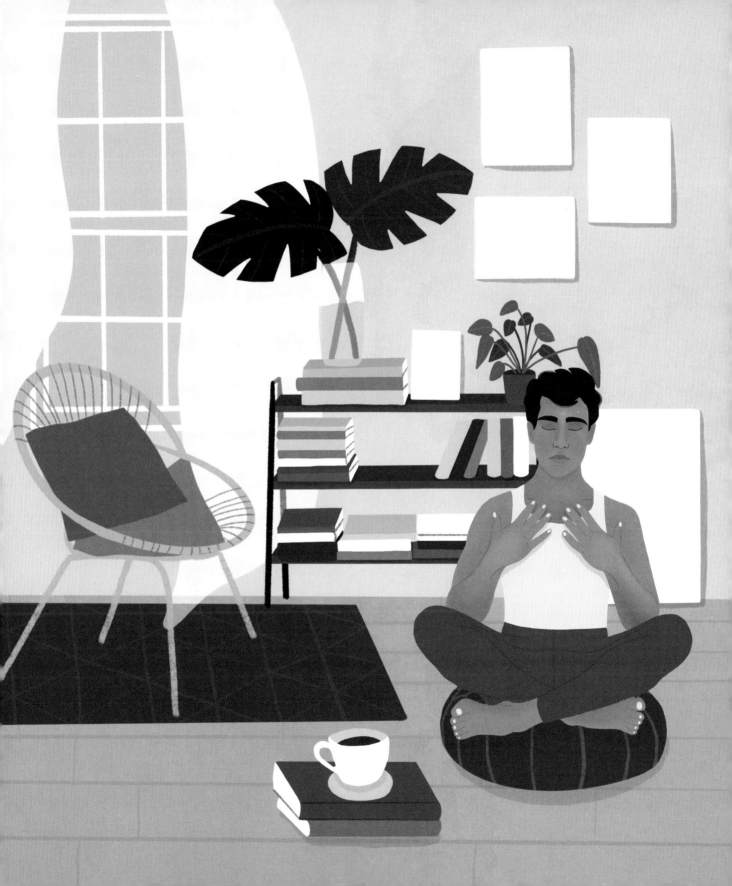

Asanas: Seated Forward Bends

ALLOW ABOUT 35 MINUTES

One of the greatest misconceptions about yoga is that it is meant to purify the body. While a strong physical practice will support the body's detoxification processes, toxins and waste products are a natural part of being human. Bringing *saucha* onto the mat is less about cleansing your body and more about purifying your mind of any toxic thoughts and judgements that prevent you from being present in your practice. This week, as we add in a series of seated forward bends, focus on practising without judgement or expectation. You might want to set an intention at the start of your practice to listen to your body and make healthy choices, both on and off the mat.

1 **Opening Sequence**
(*see p. 58*)

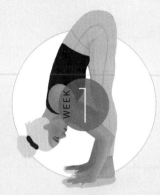

2 Repeat **WEEK 1:**
Standing Forward Bends
(*see pp. 86–7*)

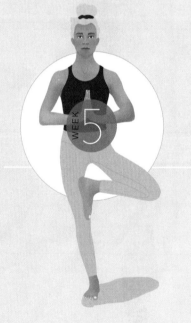

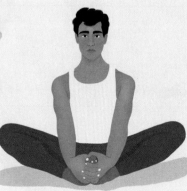

6 Repeat **WEEK 5:**
Standing Balances
(*see pp. 120–1*)

10 **Butterfly Pose**
(*see p. 136*),
5 breaths

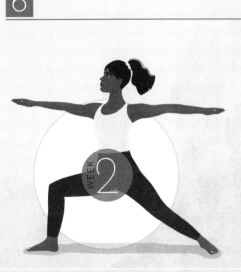

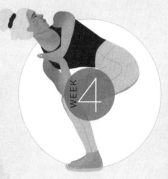

3 Repeat **WEEK 2:**
Leg-strengthening
Poses (*see pp. 94–5*)

4 Repeat **WEEK 3:**
Hip Openers and Hamstring
Stretches (*see pp. 102–3*)

5 Repeat **WEEK 4:**
Revolved Standing Poses
(*see pp. 110–11*)

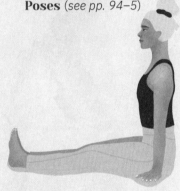

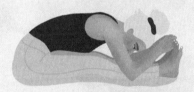

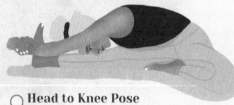

7 **Staff Pose**
(*see p. 133*),
5 breaths

8 **Seated Forward Bend**
(*see p. 134*),
5 breaths

9 **Head to Knee Pose**
(*see p. 135*),
5 breaths each side

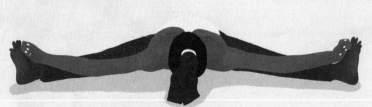

11 **Wide-legged Forward**
Bend (*see p. 137*),
5 breaths

12 **Closing Sequence**
(*see p. 75*)

Skull Shining Breath

KAPALABHATI

This is an energising, cleansing breathing practice consisting of short, powerful exhalations and passive inhalations. It is often quite challenging to begin with, so be patient as you learn to work with your breath. Make sure you practise on an empty stomach.

1 Begin in a seated position, grounding downwards through your tailbone and lengthening the crown of your head towards the sky. Cup one hand in the other and rest them gently against your lower belly.

2 Take a deep inhalation through your nose, allowing your belly to expand, and then, as if a bug flew up your nostril, exhale forcefully, pushing the air out of your lungs by contracting your lower belly inwards.

3 Immediately relax your belly and allow air to flow into your lungs so your inhalation is entirely passive.

4 Repeat this eight to ten times at a rate of one breath every second, creating a rhythm driven by the contraction and relaxation of the abdomen. After the first round, breathe naturally for a few moments and then repeat for another three to four rounds.

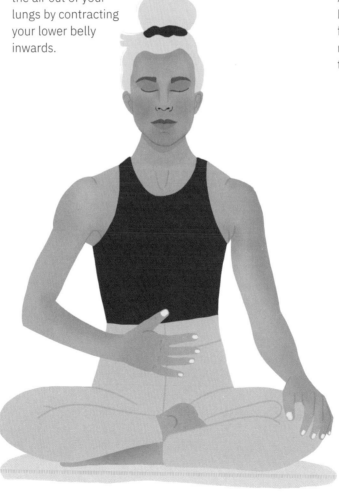

Staff Pose

DANDASANA

This is a seated version of Mountain Pose (*see* p. 64), giving you the opportunity to centre and ground yourself, and tune into your energy levels as you move through your practice.

1 Sit with your legs outstretched in front of you, either together or hip-width apart. Root down through your sitting bones, spreading them wide by rolling your thighs inwards slightly, and lift out of your pelvis, lengthening upwards through the crown of your head.

2 Pull back on your toes to flex your feet.

3 Place your hands either side of your hips and push them firmly into the ground. Lengthen the back of your neck, engaging *Jalandhara Bandha* (*see* p. 50) and gaze to the tip of your nose.

If it feels uncomfortable to sit with outstretched legs without rounding your spine, sit on the edge of a folded blanket or cushion to lift your hips slightly.

PRACTICE TIP

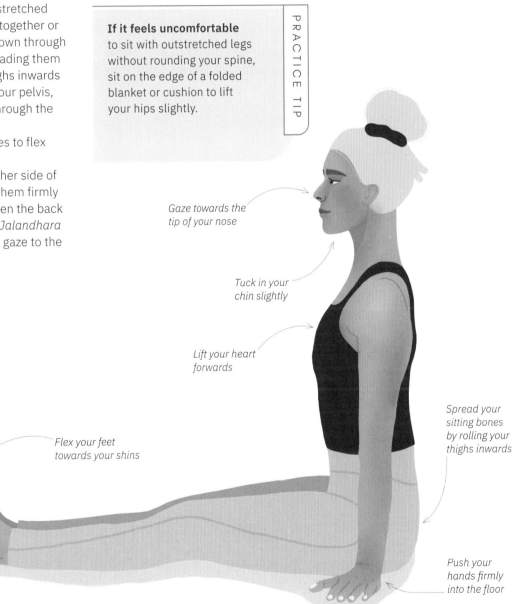

Gaze towards the tip of your nose

Tuck in your chin slightly

Lift your heart forwards

Flex your feet towards your shins

Spread your sitting bones by rolling your thighs inwards

Push your hands firmly into the floor

Seated Forward Bend

PASCHIMOTTANASANA

This is a deep forward bend, creating openness in the back of the body. If the stretch feels too intense, raise your hips on a folded blanket or cushion and thread a strap around your feet to help you fold forwards.

1 From Staff Pose (*see* p. 133), ground through your tailbone and on an inhalation, extend your arms overhead.

2 As you exhale, fold forwards, keep your arms overhead for as long as you can. When you can't fold forwards any further, bring your hands down to take hold of your shins, ankles or the outside edges of your feet or big toes. Gaze towards your toes. Or, if you're far enough down, towards the tip of your nose.

3 Create length through your spine with each inhalation. With each exhalation, release deeper into the forward bend.

4 To exit: On an inhale, lift your chest by drawing your tailbone downwards and return to Staff Pose.

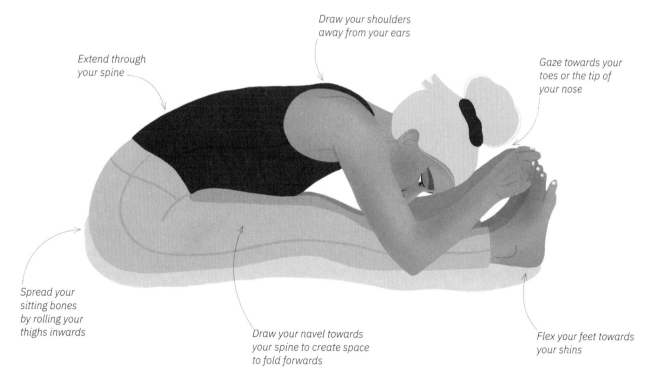

Draw your shoulders away from your ears

Extend through your spine

Gaze towards your toes or the tip of your nose

Spread your sitting bones by rolling your thighs inwards

Draw your navel towards your spine to create space to fold forwards

Flex your feet towards your shins

Head to Knee Pose

JANU SIRSASANA

This pose provides a strong stretch to the hamstring and a gentle spinal twist.
Use a strap if you struggle to reach the foot.

1 From Staff Pose (*see* p. 133), bend your left knee towards you and allow it to drop out to the side, placing the sole of your foot against your right inner thigh.

2 Align your torso to face forwards over your right leg and on an inhalation, lengthen your spine and reach your fingers towards the sky. Exhale and bow forwards, bringing your hands to rest on your shin or ankle, or taking hold of your foot. Remember that going deeper isn't always better. Focus on feeling the sensations in your body rather than making the pose look a certain way.

3 Gaze towards your outstretched foot, creating length through your spine with each inhalation, and with each exhalation releasing deeper into the forward bend.

4 To exit: On an inhale, lift your chest and lengthen out the bent leg to return to Staff Pose. Repeat on the other side.

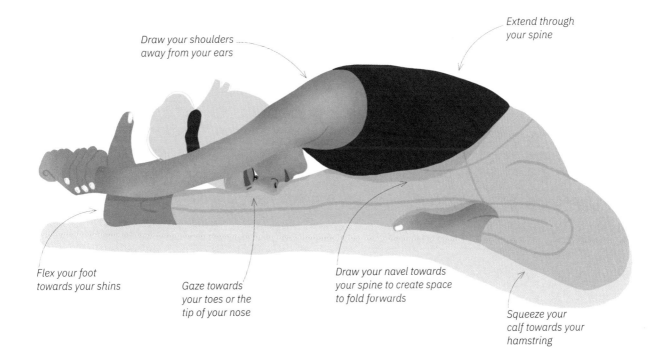

Draw your shoulders away from your ears

Extend through your spine

Flex your foot towards your shins

Gaze towards your toes or the tip of your nose

Draw your navel towards your spine to create space to fold forwards

Squeeze your calf towards your hamstring

Butterfly Pose

BADDHA KONASANA

This is also known as Bound Angle Pose. It strengthens and opens the hips and groin.

1 From Staff Pose (*see* p. 133), bend your knees and bring the soles of your feet together, drawing them towards your groin.

2 Ground through your sitting bones and lengthen the crown of your head towards the sky. Activate your glutes and squeeze your calves against your hamstrings, using your hands to gently peel the soles of your feet open like a book to help increase the rotation in your hips.

3 Gaze towards the tip of your nose, either breathing here or exploring folding forwards if that feels comfortable for you.

4 To exit: Draw your knees together and lengthen your legs out in front of you to return to Staff Pose.

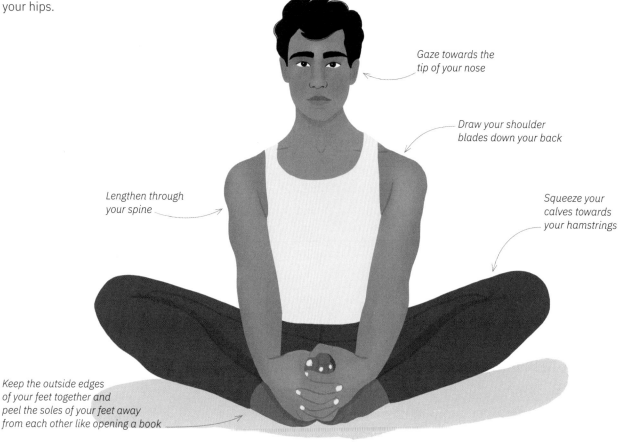

Gaze towards the tip of your nose

Draw your shoulder blades down your back

Squeeze your calves towards your hamstrings

Lengthen through your spine

Keep the outside edges of your feet together and peel the soles of your feet away from each other like opening a book

Wide-legged Forward Bend

UPAVISTHA KONASANA

Some people find this quite challenging so work with your body, sitting on a block, cushion or folded blanket to raise your hips if you need to.

1 From Staff Pose (*see p. 133*) open your legs to a V-shape, flexing your toes back towards your shins. Ground down through your sitting bones by rolling your thighs inwards so your knees face upwards towards the sky and lengthen through your spine.

2 Inhale and raise your arms above your head and, as you exhale, bow forwards, spreading your arms wide to take hold of the outside edges of your feet. If this is too intense, rest your hands on your shins or ankles.

3 Gaze towards the tip of your nose, lengthening your spine with each inhalation and drawing deeper into the pose as you exhale.

4 To exit: On an inhale, lift your chest and draw your legs together to return to Staff Pose.

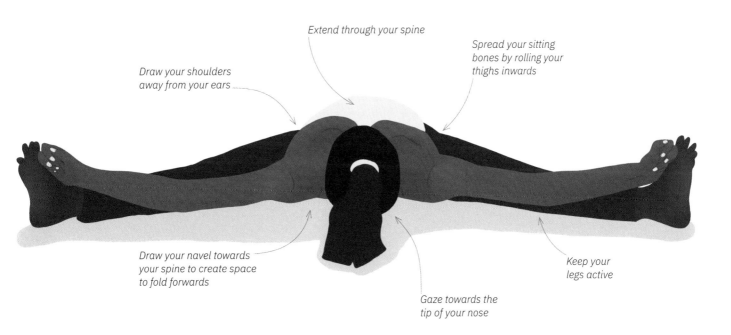

Extend through your spine

Draw your shoulders away from your ears

Spread your sitting bones by rolling your thighs inwards

Draw your navel towards your spine to create space to fold forwards

Gaze towards the tip of your nose

Keep your legs active

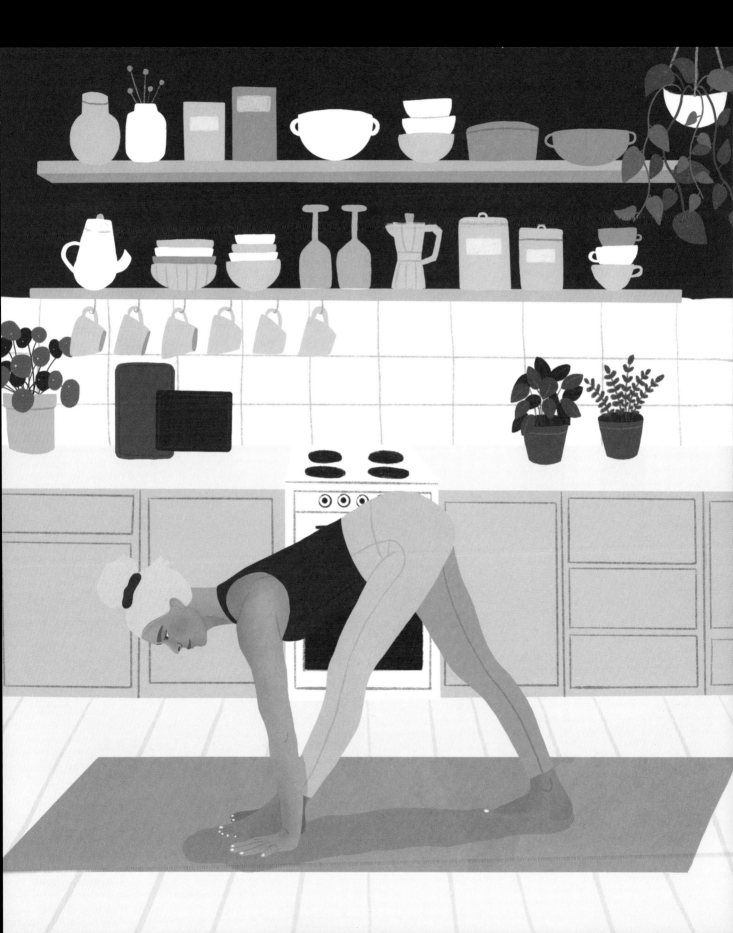

WEEK 7 Contentment

SANTOSHA

YOGA INVITES US to drop below the surface of our lives. To step off into the unknown. To walk into the shadows of ourselves. At times, it can be a fierce and challenging practice that reduces us to our most naked self. That reminds us to love whatever this life gives us. That encourages us to embrace every moment of this brief and precious adventure of being alive.

From the peaks of joy and valleys of grief to the oceans of love and dark woods of our aloneness, *santosha* is a powerful practice that reminds us how fragile it all is. How, beneath every experience, no matter how terrible, there lives a deep, spiritual joy within us; an inner peace that cannot be shaken by anything in the outside world. How everything we go through is an invitation to live more fully, love more deeply and learn how to let go.

Santosha means 'unconditional acceptance' or 'complete contentment'. It is a concept that is often rejected in the Western world of continuous progress, as if it is our discontent and unhappiness that motivates us rather than an innate longing to grow, awaken and share our gifts with the world. Being content with our lives doesn't mean idly sitting back and watching our days pass us by. Contentment isn't saying, 'My life is pretty good so I won't bother meditating or growing my own vegetables or writing that book.' Rather, it's freeing ourselves from the grass-is-always-greener trance. It's being okay with our perfectly imperfect body and relationships and lives instead of constantly thinking happiness is over there, when we get the flat stomach or new car or bigger house. It's fully accepting ourselves and our lives, as messy or mundane or magnificent as they are. And, from this place of calm contentment, we begin to see things more clearly and make conscious,

mindful choices about our lives rather than constantly striving towards goals that don't really matter to us.

In a culture that is constantly telling us that we are not enough – that we should do more, earn more, buy more, have more and be more – complete contentment is a challenging practice. Our task is to train our mind to see through our social conditioning so we no longer rely on the external things we have been taught to believe will make us happy to bring us happiness. Instead, as we practise *santosha* and let go of the self-destructive stories we have been telling ourselves – 'I'm not smart enough', 'I'm not pretty enough', 'I'm not good enough' – we begin to see ourselves differently: through the eyes of love instead of hate, acceptance instead of rejection, wholeness instead of lack. And, when we look at ourselves and the world through these eyes, we discover we have enough and we are enough. We escape the trance of unworthiness that fooled us into thinking that losing weight, or getting a promotion, or meeting the perfect partner could make us happy forever and instead realise that we can find peace and happiness right where we are.

Every single one of us has, at some point in our lives, found ourselves thinking, 'I'll be happy when I lose the weight/buy the house/get married ...'. And probably, what we discover is that when we do lose the weight/buy the house/get married, our initial happiness soon dissolves and we quickly move on to chasing the next thing we hope will make us happy, trapping us in an endless spiral of dissatisfaction and desire. In many ways the practice of *santosha* is a mindset, an attitude, a way of being in the world. It asks us to dive beneath the surface chaos of our lives and sense the deep, joyful stillness that lives beneath it. It allows us to see abundance where we previously saw scarcity, opportunity where we usually see failure, and beauty where we used to see pain. In many ways, *santosha* allows us to give ourselves fully to the goals that really matter to us because we are no longer basing our entire sense of worth and happiness on achieving them.

With time and practise, we begin to completely accept whatever life brings us. We develop the capacity to stay firmly rooted in deep inner peace even if we find our external life crumbling at our feet. We become available to the world and all its suffering because we have glimpsed a strength within us that is unshakable. We know, in the core of our being, we are strong, we are worthy, we are whole.

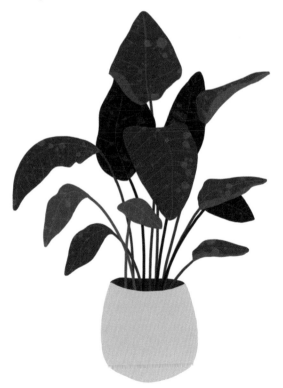

Mindful Living Practice

Many of us live with a vague emptiness, a gnawing ache of something missing, a free-floating anxiety that there is never enough – time, money, love – and so we spend our lives trying to fill this void, this hole in our soul, with external things. Capitalism fuels this message in subtle and not-so-subtle ways, promising us that if we just buy this anti-wrinkle cream or that car or those trainers, we'll finally be lovable, happy, whole. Deep down, we know this isn't true. But often, in the busyness of our lives, it's easy to forget and get sucked back into the cycle of discontent. This week, create an island of relief in the busyness of your life and use the questions below to explore the situations that trigger feelings of lack and to create daily practices that remind you of the inner peace that is always right here if you slow down enough to notice it.

> *What external things am I hoping to find happiness in?*
>
> *What goals am I chasing that don't really matter to me?*
>
> *What would it be like if I could accept my life – my body, my relationships, my financial situation – exactly as it is?*
>
> *How can I practise complete contentment and unconditional acceptance in my daily life?*

For example, when you begin to look at yourself deeply, you might discover that you are searching for happiness in a new relationship, hoping that meeting the man or woman of your dreams will be the thing that makes you feel whole. Or you might realise that your goal of losing a few kilos before you go on holiday is actually the diet industry's goal and in reality, you quite like your curves and feel more energised when you let your body be at the weight it wants to be at. Each day, you could practise unconditional acceptance of your body by thinking of one thing you appreciate about living in it before every meal to remind you of the deep joy and inner freedom that comes with seeing yourself through the eyes of love instead of judgement.

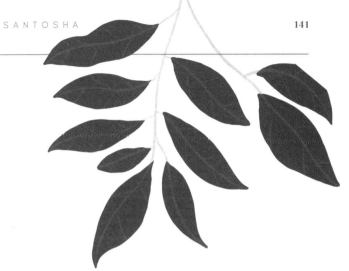

Aspiration inspiration

Cultivating *santosha* isn't always easy, especially when we are feeling unworthy or when our lives are full of difficulty or loss. Use the ideas below to inspire you to create aspirations that will help you remember the bottomless strength and boundless love that lives within you.

'May I meet each difficulty with compassion.'

'May I trust everything I need is within me.'

'May I accept myself completely.'

Look for beauty

If we have spent a long time living from a place of lack and discontent, always seeing what is wrong with ourselves and the world, we need to train our mind to look for beauty. This is a conscious practice that reawakens us to the simple joys that are around us every moment and reminds us that the world is a wonderful place. This week, pause every hour or two and find one thing that is beautiful in that moment; something that fills you with wonder and awe. Usually these things look a lot like ordinary life: the cute dog in the coffee shop, the pattern of the clouds, the way your socks hug your ankles, the elderly couple holding hands, the sound of the zip on your coat. Beauty hides in the most unusual places. We simply have to open our eyes and look for it.

Meditation

Loving-Kindness (*metta*) Meditation

Contentment is the capacity to love what is. This isn't always easy. Meditation gives us an opportunity to cultivate an unconditional acceptance, love and compassion for whatever we are going through, whomever we meet and whoever we are. And, as we become more embodied through our practice, we begin to notice the pure joy that flows through us when we say yes to life; when we learn to love it all; when we accept the sacred messiness of being alive.

Loving-Kindness Meditation is a gentle but powerful practice that enables us to cultivate loving acceptance for ourselves and others. As we practise, our hearts begin to open and we start to feel compassion for all living beings, even those whom we may be prejudiced against or whom we feel have wronged us. We develop the inner strength to let another's suffering touch our heart and wish for them to be free from it.

You can practise Loving-Kindness Meditation for anywhere from five minutes to one hour, combining it with other meditation techniques if you wish. Begin in your seated meditation position and close your eyes. Cultivate a feeling of compassion – of unconditional acceptance, of loving-kindness, of cherishing – for yourself – and silently say, 'May I be happy and free from suffering.' After a couple of minutes, widen your circle of compassion to include someone you love and silently wish for them to be happy and free from suffering: 'May you be happy and free from suffering.' Again, after a few minutes, expand your circle of loving-kindness further to include someone you don't know very well – a neighbour, your postman, a barista in the coffee shop down the road – and wish that they too are happy and free from suffering. Extend your circle of compassion once more, this time to include someone you find difficult or don't like. Feel loving kindness ripple through you as you wish them happiness and to be free from suffering. Then take a moment to feel loving kindness for all of the above people at once. Finally, let this loving kindness flow out to all living beings: 'May all beings in the world be happy and free.'

Some people find it very difficult to begin cultivating loving kindness for themselves, so if you are struggling, start by cultivating it for someone you love deeply – a friend, a child, a partner, a parent, even a pet – and then expand your circle of loving kindness to include yourself.

Asanas: Seated Twists

ALLOW ABOUT 40 MINUTES

Our time on the mat is a beautiful place to explore what it is like to live with complete acceptance. The poses give us an opportunity to appreciate how far we have come and accept where we are in our physical practice, even if we can't do everything we'd like to be able to do yet. By letting go of the need to be stronger or more flexible and simply accepting where our body is now, we experience the freedom that comes with no longer striving for perfection and simply trusting that wherever we are is exactly where we need to be. This week, we add in a series of seated twists, so as you practise, take a moment to remind yourself there is no deadline when it comes to yoga. There is nothing to prove or achieve. And the more we practise from a place of acceptance, the more we can experience the beauty of being exactly where we are right now.

1 Opening Sequence
(see p. 58)

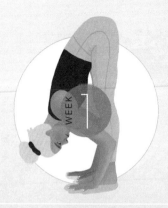

2 Repeat WEEK 1:
Standing Forward Bends
(see pp. 86–7)

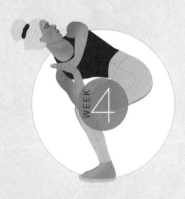

5 Repeat WEEK 4:
Revolved Standing Poses
(see pp. 110–11)

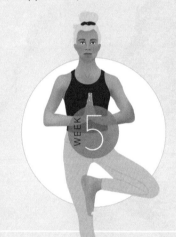

6 Repeat
WEEK 5:
**Standing
Balances**
(see pp. 120–1)

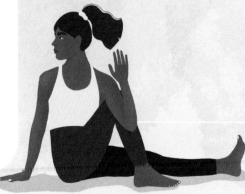

10 Seated Twist
(see p. 145), 5 breaths
then transition to
next pose

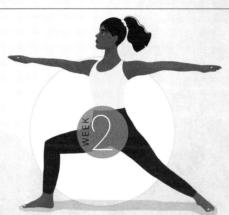

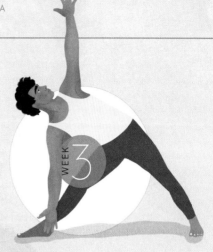

3 Repeat **WEEK 2:**
Leg-strengthening Poses
(*see pp. 94–5*)

4 Repeat **WEEK 3:**
Hip Openers and Hamstring Stretches
(*see pp. 102–3*)

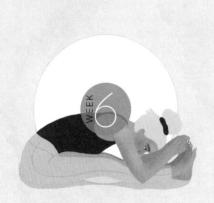

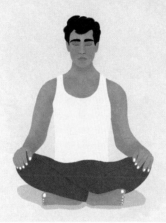

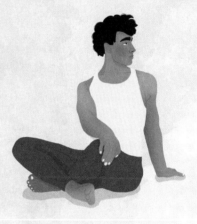

7 Repeat **WEEK 6:**
Seated Forward Bends
(*see pp. 130–1*)

8 **Easy Pose**
(*see p. 80*),
5 breaths

9 **Easy Twist**
(*see p. 144*),
5 breaths each side

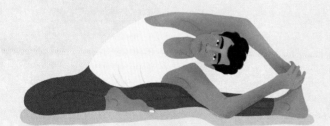

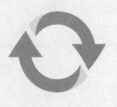

11 **Revolved Head to Knee Pose**
(*see p. 146*), 5 breaths each side

12 **Repeat poses
10 and 11** on the
other side

13 **Closing Sequence**
(*see p. 75*)

Easy Twist

PRARIVRTTA SUKHASANA

Gentle spinal twists such as this one help to maintain spinal mobility and support the health of discs and joints.

1 Begin in Easy Pose (*see* p. 80), rooting down through your sitting bones. Inhale and reach your arms to the sky.

2 On an exhale, rotate to your right, bringing your left hand down to land on your right knee and placing your right hand down behind you. Gaze backwards over your right shoulder.

3 Work with your breath, creating length in your spine as you inhale, and gently increasing the rotation as you exhale.

4 To exit: On an inhale, reach your arms overhead and return to centre. As you exhale repeat the twist on the other side.

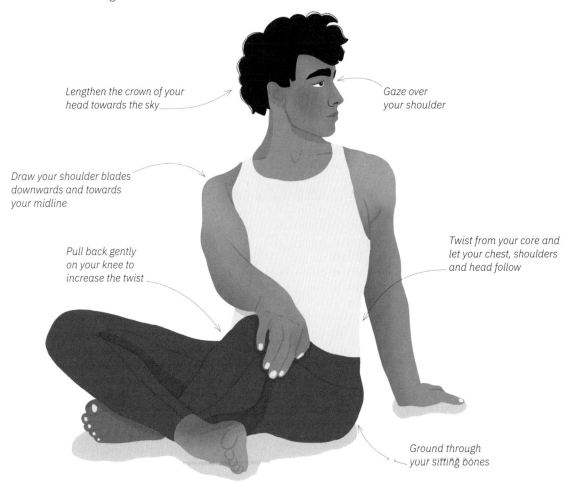

Lengthen the crown of your head towards the sky

Gaze over your shoulder

Draw your shoulder blades downwards and towards your midline

Pull back gently on your knee to increase the twist

Twist from your core and let your chest, shoulders and head follow

Ground through your sitting bones

Seated Twist

MARICHYASANA C

A gentle twist for relieving tension in the spine.

1 Begin in Staff Pose (*see* p. 133) and draw your right knee in towards your chest, placing your foot about a fist's distance away from your inner thigh. Flex the toes of your left foot towards the sky.

2 Reach your right arm behind you and as you inhale, lengthen your left arm to the sky. As you exhale, twist towards your right leg, bending your left elbow and bringing it to the outside of your right thigh.

3 Create length in your spine by pushing your right hand firmly into the floor and with each exhalation, gently twist deeper into the pose, twisting from your waist and gazing back over your right shoulder.

4 To exit: On an inhale, rotate back to centre and as you exhale, lower your right knee to the side so your outer thigh is on the ground, preparing for Revolved Head to Knee Pose (*see* p. 146). If you aren't following the sequence in the book, simply lengthen your right leg out to return to Staff Pose before repeating on the other side.

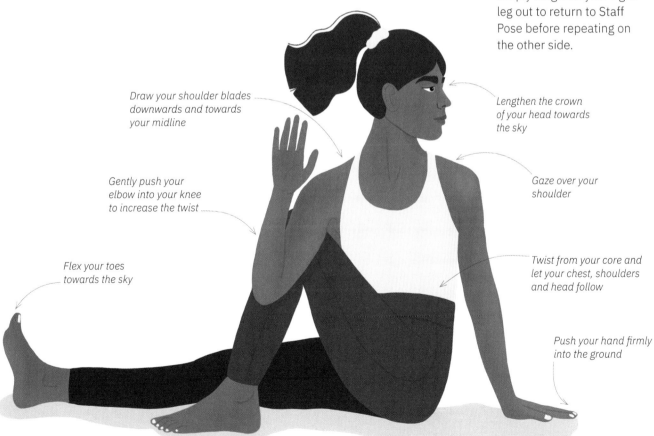

Draw your shoulder blades downwards and towards your midline

Lengthen the crown of your head towards the sky

Gently push your elbow into your knee to increase the twist

Gaze over your shoulder

Flex your toes towards the sky

Twist from your core and let your chest, shoulders and head follow

Push your hand firmly into the ground

Revolved Head to Knee Pose

PARIVRITTA JANU SIRSASANA

This pose offers a beautiful stretch to the side of the body while creating openness through the chest. Use the outstretched leg as your anchor.

1 From Staff Pose (*see* p. 133) draw your right leg into your chest and let it fall out to the side, creating a 90-degree angle at your groin.

2 Rotate your torso so it's facing the space between your legs and lean sideways over your left leg, bringing your left forearm to rest on your left thigh or on the ground just inside your shin. Extend your right arm overhead, gaze upwards towards your right fingers and rotate your chest towards the sky.

3 For a deeper stretch, reach your right hand all the way over to take hold of the outside of your left foot, making sure your chest doesn't collapse inwards.

4 To exit: On an inhale, lift your chest back to centre and release your arms by your side. Lengthen your right leg out to return to Staff Pose and repeat on the other side.

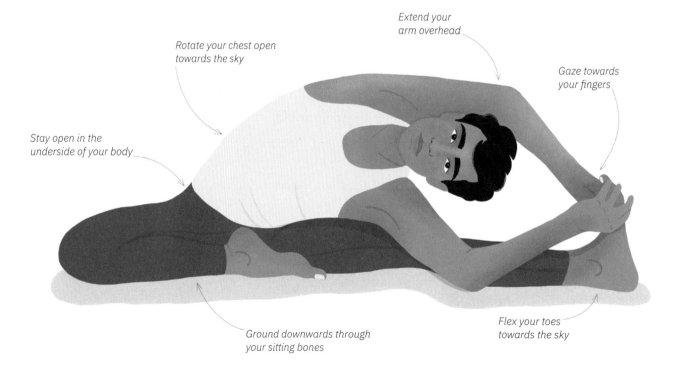

Rotate your chest open towards the sky

Extend your arm overhead

Gaze towards your fingers

Stay open in the underside of your body

Ground downwards through your sitting bones

Flex your toes towards the sky

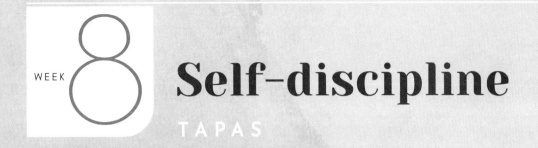

8

Self-discipline

TAPAS

THROUGH OUR PRACTICE, yoga gifts us with a fierce and undying devotion to the world. Each time we step on our mat instead of lounging on the sofa, or sit in meditation instead of mindlessly scrolling through our phone, or choose to face our vulnerable feelings instead of running from them, we stoke the fire of transformation within us. We cultivate the loving discipline required to remember our wholeness and reclaim the fullness of our power.

Tapas is our inner fire. It is the willingness to do the work. It is our commitment to health and wholeness. It is the discipline, dedication and devotion we bring to our practice, our relationships and our lives. This self-discipline is never self-destructive. It is always directed towards wholeness; to building a healthy body, cultivating a clear mind and awakening the dormant energy within that fills us with aliveness. On a practical level, *tapas* might include creating a better sleep pattern – turning off technology in the evening and going to bed an hour earlier – or adopting a healthier diet and committing to a daily walk on our lunch break.

Creating these healthy habits isn't always easy. As humans, we don't like change and even when we know the changes we are making will lead to greater health and happiness, we often experience a lot of resistance to making them. It is the practice of *tapas* that ensures we follow through on the promises we make to ourselves. We need this inner fire to fuel us through the procrastination, inertia and discomfort that we will experience as we begin changing the deeply rooted habits that are causing us unease, poor health and dissatisfaction with life. As we apply the fiery determination of tapas to our daily lives – in the changes we need to make and the challenges we need to overcome – we are transformed by it. Our

discipline and dedication shapes us into stronger, kinder, more devoted human beings.

Rather than force or willpower, *tapas* is rooted in a deep love for our practice, an emotional clarity about our values, actions and goals, and a loving commitment to our journey towards wholeness. This self-discipline needs to include self-compassion if we are to transform our most destructive and deep-rooted habits into tools for awakening. Because, as we release old habits, there will be days when we stumble and slip back into ingrained ways of thinking and behaving. Without this compassion, we simply find ourselves in a cycle of shame and blame, treating ourselves as a never-ending self-improvement project.

As we bring the practice of *tapas* into our lives, it is helpful to remind ourselves that yoga is not a quest to become a better and better human. Rather, it is a practice in becoming fully human. *Tapas* is the fire deep within us that, when cultivated, burns away everything we are not, everything that is hiding our true Self. It pushes our mind against its own limits: our destructive thought patterns, unrealistic expectations and limiting beliefs. It asks us to hold on, to hold out, for healing, for love, for life. It gives us the strength to stay with our fear, our grief, our frustration, while our suffering is transformed into something beautiful and sacred.

Tapas breaks us open to an inner power we may have forgotten existed. A fierce and gentle power that has been hiding beneath our self-doubt and insecurity all along. A transformational power that awakens us to a vast freedom, a deep trust, a glittering aliveness. A power that gives us the courage to share the gifts we carry for the world.

Mindful Living Practice

Journal prompts

It's so easy to get caught up in our daily routines that it's only when we pause and look inwards we realise the ways in which we have been living on autopilot and fallen into unhealthy habits. Often, we know what we need to do: eat more fruit, drink more water, drink less wine, quit smoking, go to the gym, spend more time with our parents, go to bed earlier. But we don't do it. Sometimes out of ignorance, sometimes out of exhaustion, but mostly out of fear – of failure, of discomfort, of change. And sometimes, it is our fear of surrender that keeps us imprisoned in habits that are taking us out of balance. Our self-discipline is no longer loving but regimented, harsh, destructive. Use the questions below to reflect on areas of your life that require more self-discipline to bring you back to wholeness and where it would be more nourishing to release control and allow space for intuition, spontaneity and surrender.

Where am I lacking self-discipline in my life?

Where has my self-discipline tipped over into deprivation and obsession?

How can I practise loving discipline in my daily life?

For example, you may realise that you need to get to sleep by ten o'clock in order to get the eight hours rest that leave you feeling your best. Here, *tapas* might look like setting yourself a bedtime alarm as a reminder to get ready for bed. Or, you might realise that you are lacking discipline in your meditation practice so self-discipline could mean asking your partner to remind you to meditate after dinner every night (or even asking them to meditate with you.)

Aspiration inspiration

At times, we all lose touch with our inner fire. We feel disempowered, uninspired and full of doubt. We find ourselves giving up before we have even begun. The words we speak to ourselves can act as sparks that reignite the fire within us. That remind us of our passion, our power, our capacity to grow and change and make a difference to the world. Use the ideas below to inspire your own aspirations to cultivate *tapas* and invite self-belief, self-compassion and self-discipline into your life.

'May my inner fire be ignited.'

'May I choose loving discipline over harsh restraint.'

'When I fall, may I get back up again. Stronger, braver and more loving.'

One tiny promise

Whatever we think or do repeatedly becomes a habit, a pathway in the brain that influences our thoughts and actions in the future. If we regularly make tiny promises to ourselves – to eat better or go to bed earlier or start a meditation practice – and follow through, our mind learns that we can trust ourselves to do what we say we are going to do. If we regularly practise yoga first thing in the morning, our mind and body are primed to get on our mat as soon as we wake up. And, if we regularly focus on how we can help others, our mind and heart opens to all the tiny, humble opportunities for kindness that show up in our daily lives.

We can embrace the power of *tapas* to release thought and behavioural patterns that are taking us away from health and wholeness and to create conscious habits that are in alignment with our values. These changes don't need to be grand or fantastical. And we certainly don't need to overhaul our entire lives. In fact, a small change approach has been found to be far more successful in everything from weight loss to professional development.

This week, bring your awareness to any thought patterns or behavioural habits that are having a negative effect on your health and happiness and focus on making one small change in your personal or professional life: one tiny promise to yourself that you know you can stick to. If you would like to feel more connected to your partner, it could be as simple as spending five minutes with them when you get in from work – fully present and fully alive – instead of rushing to do the chores straight away. If you often find yourself trapped in the never-enough trance, it could be saying 'thank you' as soon as you wake up in the morning to celebrate the sheer joy of being alive. Or, if you feel addicted to your phone, it could be initiating a no-phone rule between seven o'clock in the evening and seven o'clock in the morning.

Breathwork – *pranayama*

Pranayama is a beautiful way to cultivate *tapas* and challenge our habitual way of breathing to help quieten our mind. By regulating our breath, we regulate our mind. If one is steady, the other is steady too. As our breath steadies, our awareness deepens and we invite our subconscious thoughts, stored emotions and limiting beliefs to the surface, where we can set them free. As we release these limiting beliefs, we realise our potential and tap into our power.

Skull Shining Breath (*see* p. 132) is often practised to ignite the inner fire of *tapas* and burn away these limiting beliefs and everything we are not.

Square Breathing – involving breath retention as well as lengthening of the inhalation and exhalation – is another powerful *pranayama* that allows the mind to quieten, our awareness to deepen and our determination and discipline to strengthen. You might like to practise Square Breathing before you meditate to steady your mind, or at any other time of day when you are feeling disempowered, your inner critic is filling your mind with excuses and self-doubt, or you find yourself procrastinating or lacking discipline. You can find full instructions on page 152.

Meditation

Tonglen Meditation

It takes discipline to stay true to our values when we are suffering. Tonglen Meditation – which means 'accepting and sending out' – is one of the most powerful practices of compassion that helps us to be with own emotional suffering and open our hearts to the pain of others. Using our breath, our intentions and our imagination, we cultivate the capacity to stay present with difficult feelings both on the meditation cushion and when we experience pain, resistance or suffering – our own or others' – in our daily lives.

Begin in your meditation posture and close your eyes. If you feel ungrounded, use Loving Awareness Meditation (*see* p. 101), Earth Breathing (*see* p. 118–9) or Ten-point Meditation (*see* p. 128) to help centre you. Set an intention to stay present with whatever suffering arises and, as you did when practising Loving-Kindness Meditation (*see* p. 141) connect with your compassion, your soft spot. Some people find it helpful to bring to mind a time in their life when they have felt unconditionally loved or imagine themselves being showered in an endless, wholehearted love. Stay connected to this deep source of love and compassion and at the same time, bring your awareness to the suffering in the world, visualising it as black smog. As you inhale, imagine yourself breathing in this dark, polluted smoke, this general feeling of negativity or suffering. Hold this smog inside for a moment, feel it transform in the light of love you are connected to and, as you exhale, imagine yourself breathing out, fresh, pure, bright air. As you inhale, you are 'accepting' the polluted smoke, and as you exhale, you are 'sending out' the clean, nourishing air. Do this for a minute or two.

Now bring to mind someone in your life who is struggling or suffering in some way and visualise the difficulties in their life as smoky dark clouds. Without fear, breathe in the dark clouds of their suffering, holding your breath for just a moment as this suffering is transformed through the compassion in your heart, and, as you exhale, imagine yourself breathing out a healing, white light full of peace, love, joy or whatever this person needs. Do this for as long as you need.

You may like to move on to someone else who is suffering, or a group of people who are struggling, repeating the process of breathing in the black smoke of suffering, feeling it transform into the healing these people need inside you and then breathing out this pure, nourishing light of healing as you exhale. Breathe in suffering. Transform. Breathe out healing.

You may also like to devote some time in your practice to your own healing. Inhaling the pain you are feeling – physically or emotionally – holding it in your heart for a moment and then breathing out compassion, tenderness and healing to wherever needs it.

Asanas: Arm Balances

ALLOW 40-45 MINUTES

Our time on the mat is one of the most powerful ways to cultivate and practise *tapas*. This week includes a series of arm balances that can feel as terrifying as they do empowering. As we practise these more challenging poses, we *will* fall out of them. This gives us an opportunity to ride the waves of fear and failure and invites us to be disciplined in practising those poses we find particularly difficult. This week, commit to practising the arm balances – and any other poses you feel resistance to – consistently. You might want to commit to practising each pose three times or playing with each pose until you have fallen out of it five times. This gives you the opportunity to work through adversity and develop the inner fire and mental strength to keep going, to learn from each stumble, to bravely and courageously fail forwards.

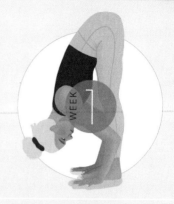

1 **Opening Sequence**
(*see p. 58*)

2 Repeat **WEEK 1:**
Standing Forward Bends
(*see pp. 86–7*)

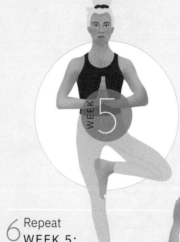

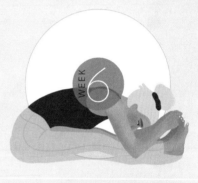

6 Repeat
WEEK 5:
Standing
Balances
(*see pp. 120–1*)

7 Repeat **WEEK 6:**
Seated Forward Bends
(*see pp. 130–1*)

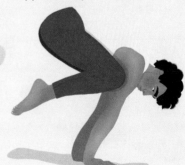

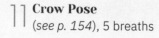

10 **Side Plank Pose** or
Gate Pose (*see p. 153*),
5 breaths each side

11 **Crow Pose**
(*see p. 154*), 5 breaths

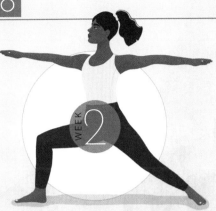

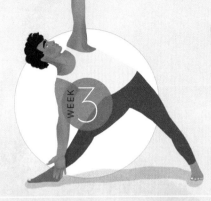

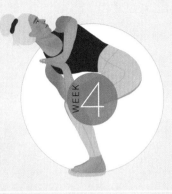

3 Repeat **WEEK 2:**
Leg Strengthening Poses
(*see pp. 94–5*)

4 Repeat **WEEK 3:**
Hip Openers and Hamstring Stretches (*see pp. 102–3*)

5 Repeat **WEEK 4:**
Revolved Standing Poses
(*see pp. 110–11*)

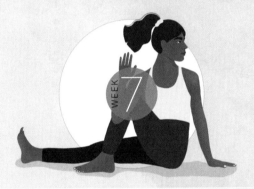

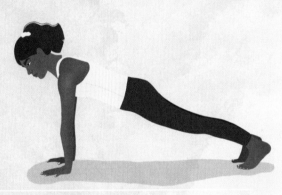

8 Repeat **WEEK 7:**
Seated Twists (*see pp. 142–3*)

9 **Plank Pose**
(*see p. 68*), 5 breaths

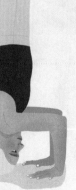

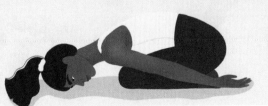

12 **Tripod Headstand**
(*see p. 155*),
5 breaths

13 **Child's Pose**
(*see p. 156*),
20 breaths

14 **Closing Sequence**
(*see p. 75*)

Square Breathing
SAMA VRITTI

This is a variation of Equal Breathing (*see* p. 62), which includes a pause at the top of the inhalation and bottom of the exhalation, creating a sense of calm and grounding.

1 Sit in Easy Pose (*see* p. 80). Breathing in and out through your nose, establish a rhythm where your inhalation and exhalation become four counts each.

2 Add in a pause at the top of your inhalation and the bottom of your exhalation the same length as the inhalation and exhalation so that you are breathing in for a count of four, holding for a count of four, exhaling for a count of four and holding your exhalation for a count of four.

3 Repeat for five to ten rounds.

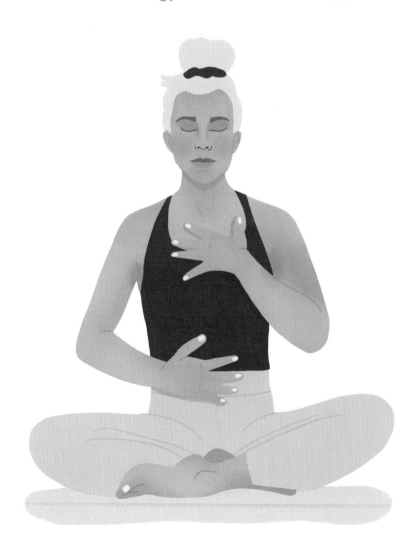

Side Plank Pose

VASISTHASANA

This is a strong pose that builds strength in your shoulders, core and side body. If it feels too strong or your body is feeling tired, practise Gate Pose (*see* variation) as a gentler alternative.

1 From Plank Pose (*see* p. 68), place your right hand towards the centre of the mat and let your heels fall to the right, resting on the outside of your right foot and stacking your left foot on top of your right.

2 Push your right hand firmly into the ground and lift your left hand, either resting it on your left thigh or reaching it towards the sky, helping to open the entire front of your body sideways.

3 Stabilise through your right shoulder by wrapping your triceps under. Try not to lock the elbow. Squeeze your knees together to keep your core stable and lengthen your tailbone towards your heels, making sure your pelvis doesn't sag. Gaze straight ahead or towards your top hand.

4 To exit: Lower your top hand to the floor to return to Plank Pose and repeat on the other side.

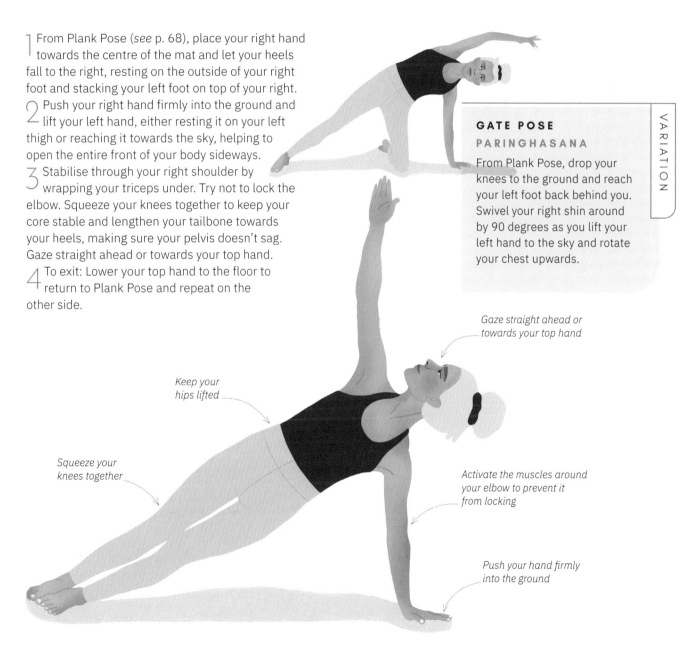

VARIATION

GATE POSE
PARINGHASANA

From Plank Pose, drop your knees to the ground and reach your left foot back behind you. Swivel your right shin around by 90 degrees as you lift your left hand to the sky and rotate your chest upwards.

Gaze straight ahead or towards your top hand

Keep your hips lifted

Squeeze your knees together

Activate the muscles around your elbow to prevent it from locking

Push your hand firmly into the ground

Crow Pose

BAKASANA

This is a challenging arm balance so approach it with an attitude of play. You can place a couple of cushions in front of you to create a sense of safety if you feel afraid of falling.

1 From a squat position, place your hands on the mat, shoulder-width apart and spread your fingers wide to create a strong base.

2 Lean your torso forwards, lifting your sitting bones high enough to snuggle your knees in towards your armpits and rest your shins on the backs of your upper arms.

3 Come up onto the balls of your feet and lean forwards even more, shifting as much of your weight as possible into your hands. Either one at a time, or both together, draw your heels towards your tailbone to lift your feet off the floor. Gaze between your thumbs or to the tip of your nose. As you get more confident in this pose, see if you can begin to straighten your arms (this often takes years of practice!).

4 To exit: Simply lower your feet to the floor and take a rest if you need to.

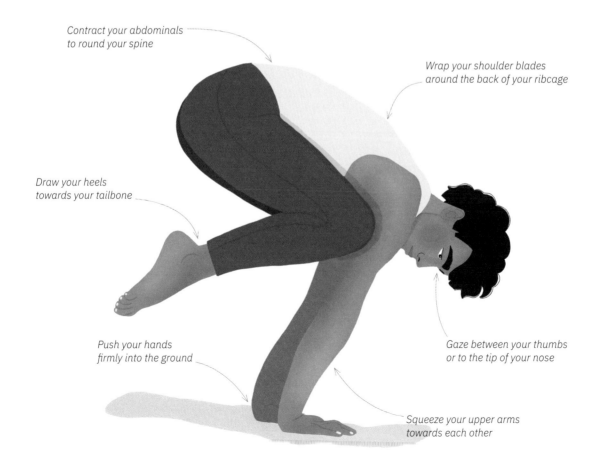

Contract your abdominals to round your spine

Wrap your shoulder blades around the back of your ribcage

Draw your heels towards your tailbone

Push your hands firmly into the ground

Gaze between your thumbs or to the tip of your nose

Squeeze your upper arms towards each other

Tripod Headstand

SIRSASANA

This is a powerful inversion. If you feel at all unsure about it, use a wall for support or save this pose for practising in class with the help of a teacher. Avoid this pose if you have any neck issues.

1 Begin on your hands and knees and lower your head to the floor about a hand's distance in front of your fingertips so your elbows are at a right angle.

2 Push your hands firmly into the ground and straighten your legs. Begin to walk your toes towards you until your hips are stacked over your shoulders. Stay here if this feels intense enough for you or step your knees onto your upper arms and squeeze your knees towards your bottom (I like to call this variation Egg Stand because the shape of the body in this pose resembles an egg!).

3 When you feel stable, begin to extend your legs straight upwards towards the sky. Point your toes, squeeze your knees together and activate your core to create stability.

4 To exit: You want to exit the pose the same way you entered it, bending your knees and lowering down with control — either bringing your knees to your upper arms or lowering your toes to the floor gracefully and with control.

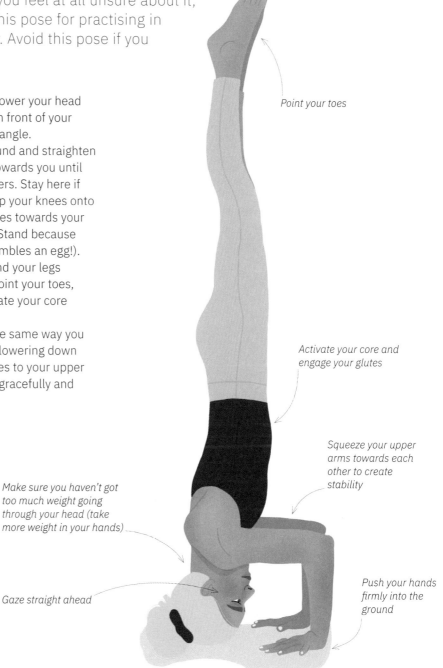

Point your toes

Activate your core and engage your glutes

Squeeze your upper arms towards each other to create stability

Make sure you haven't got too much weight going through your head (take more weight in your hands)

Push your hands firmly into the ground

Gaze straight ahead

Child's Pose

BALASANA

This is a calming, restorative pose to practise after inversions or when you notice your breath becoming fast and messy. Simply stay in this pose until your breath has returned to its natural rhythm.

1 From all fours, sit back into your heels and rest your forehead on the mat wherever is comfortable. Adjust the width of your knees if you need to or place a blanket underneath them if you notice any discomfort.

2 Either reach your arms overhead or wrap them back towards your heels, letting your shoulders fall forwards.

3 Soften your jaw, relax your breathing and let your body surrender into the pose.

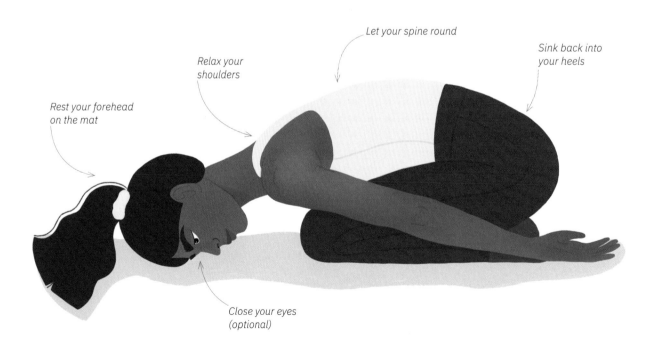

Let your spine round

Relax your shoulders

Sink back into your heels

Rest your forehead on the mat

Close your eyes (optional)

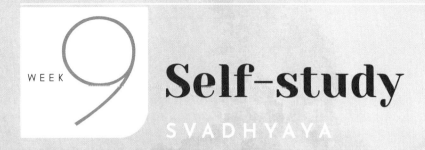

WEEK

9 Self-study

SVADHYAYA

YOGA IS AN INVITATION to discover who we really are – beneath the masks we wear, behind the walls we build, beyond the trance of unworthiness – so that we can live with greater courage, compassion and clarity because we know, deep in our bones, we are not in this world alone. We are all one. We are all whole.

Svadhyaya is the process of studying and discovering the Self. Not the small self or the ego or the person we often take ourselves to be – that busy, anxious, little 'I' so caught up with chasing goals and proving its worth and striving for more. But the vastly deeper and more authentic Self we discover when we drop beneath the surface of our lives.

The practice of reflecting on ourselves (who we are, where we come from, why we are here, how we can serve and whether we are living the life we really want to live), *svadhyaya* enables us to begin to differentiate between our ego and our true Self. By studying ourselves in this way, we become more aware of when our ego – the scared, small self – is in control and how it may be harming us. When we listen to the ego, we often find ourselves caught in a cycle of comparison and judgement. We may catch ourselves acting in ways that are not in alignment with our true values. And we are often so concerned with getting our own way or proving that we are right – usually out of insecurity and unworthiness – that we accidentally cause harm to ourselves and others.

But, the ego is not the enemy. It is simply unconscious, reactive and immature. It runs on false beliefs and outdated emotional and behavioural patterns that were programmed when we were children. And

it continues to run on them even if those patterns are causing us to suffer. It keeps us living on autopilot. Therefore, *svadhyaya* is not about destroying the ego but integrating it; developing a relationship with it where it serves us instead of one where we live as its slave. In studying ourselves, we begin to untangle our ego-based habits and the superficial identities that keep us trapped in our small self from who we really are. This self-awareness empowers us to develop healthy ego functions so we can learn from our mistakes, prioritise what will lead to long-term health and happiness, and align our inner purpose – to awaken to who we really are – with our outer purpose in the world.

In the *Yoga Sutras*, it is written: 'Study thy self, discover the divine.' In this way, *svadhyaya* is less about analysing our thoughts and emotions – as psychologists and psychiatrists do – and more about reading, writing, dancing, drumming, painting and practising anything that reconnects us with our true Self and allows us to experience the 'divine' spark that lives within all of us. This sacred spark – our Buddha nature, our inner guru, our inherent goodness – is the incorruptible part of ourselves. The unbreakable part. The unshatterable part. The part of ourselves that no pain or suffering or evil can destroy. The part of ourselves that, when rekindled and reawakened, manifests in our quest for meaning, our sense of belonging and worthiness, our desire to be of service, our search for truth and beauty, our intuitive knowing of right from wrong, and our feelings of joy, love and aliveness.

In the modern Western world, the idea of us possessing a 'divine spark' – a shared divinity, a oneness, a universal consciousness – can be a challenging concept to get our head around because science and medical advances mean that most of us see ourselves as nothing more than a physical body; an isolated, independent flesh robot. But it is the discovery of this omnipresent Self – the One dwelling in many – that *svadhyaya* helps us to realise. It is the practice of contemplating how we are the same being looking at the world through different eyes, simultaneously embracing ourselves as an individual wave and the universal ocean. In many ways, our interconnectedness has to be experienced directly rather than intellectualised. Buddhist meditation teacher Achaan Chah famously said, 'If you try to understand it intellectually, your head will probably explode.'

Another sacred verse that captures *svadhyaya* beautifully is a famous translation from the *Bhagavad Gita*: 'Yoga is the journey of the self, through the self, to the self.' On a practical level, this means experiencing and remembering our true Self. This often occurs through the reading of ancient scripture that inspire freedom – the *Bhagavad Gita*, the *Yoga Sutras*, the *Upanishads* – or any uplifting texts that awaken a feeling of belonging and aliveness within you. This could be poetry, books from spiritual teachers, or simply a line in a song that reminds you how all humans experience the things you thought you were going through alone. I have included a list of resources that have awakened me to this feeling of love, belonging, connection and freedom on page 188.

Often times, what we most need to discover about ourselves will be found where we least want to look. In the dark and dusty corners of our soul where we have hidden the emotions we don't want to feel and the parts of ourselves that bring us shame. *Svadhyaya* means shining a light on these shadowed places, knowing that all humans experience these things and that we are not alone in our fear or pain or shame. This takes courage and compassion, which is why the practice of *svadhyaya* requires us to remember the other pillars

of mindful living too, especially *ahimsa* (non-harm), *satya* (honesty), *tapas* (discipline) and *santosha* (complete acceptance).

Ultimately, yoga is the exploration of the mountains and valleys and oceans of our inner world, arriving back where we started, knowing ourselves for the first time.

Mindful Living Practice
Journal prompts

In many ways, we have been practising *svadhyaya* from the beginning of this ten-week journey. Our journal, like our yoga mat and meditation cushion, offers a space for self-discovery. A place where we can take off our masks and explore who we really are. Use the questions below to look at yourself on a deeper level so you can move closer to your true Self.

Who am I not?

Who am I?

What am I refusing to see about myself?

What am I unwilling to feel?

How can I practise self-study in my daily life?

What follows the words 'I am' often determines what we think, how we act and who we become. For example, you might realise you have spent most of your life with the story, 'I am a victim' – powerless to life's circumstances – when in reality, you are a creator and *you* get to choose the kind of life you want to live. Or you might discover that you identify yourself as a rescuer, putting everyone's needs before your own, when what you really need is for someone to hold space for you to do your own healing. As we realise who we are not – the fighter, the martyr, the hero – we are able to let go of those identities that no longer serve us, sometimes with grace and sometimes with hard work and sadness, and simply abide in the unknown.

Maybe, like me, you will never be able to answer the question, 'Who am I?', in any kind of definitive way (the best answer I have come up with is simply, 'I am'). Oftentimes, we can't capture our true Self in words,

But, when we touch it, we recognise it. Because, maybe for the first time, we feel whole. We feel deeply at peace and fully alive. We feel that finally, we are home.

Aspiration inspiration

As humans, we regularly forget who we are and get lost in the busyness of the world. *Svadhyaya* is a lifetime practice. A continuous remembering of who we are. A coming home to ourselves again and again. This week, create aspirations that will remind you of your true Self each time you get lost. You can use the aspirations below as inspiration.

'May I find myself when I get lost.'

'May I have the courage to explore the dark and dusty places in my soul and welcome them so I can feel whole.'

'In the city of my heart, may I find my home.'

Intention reflection

We don't have to limit the practise of *svadhyaya* to our journal or yoga mat. In fact, the ordinary moments of daily life – waiting in line at the supermarket, commuting to work, feeding our pets – give us the opportunity to get to know when we are living on autopilot, from a habitual or ego-based place, and when we are listening to our true Self. This week, begin to ask yourself, 'Why am I doing what I'm doing?' and 'Will this lead to long-term health and happiness?' It might work to ask yourself this every hour on the hour, or when you transition from one activity to the next, or when you feel a tightening in your stomach or a heaviness in your chest that is the body's way of communicating you might be living out of alignment with your values.

Questioning ourselves like this allows us to step back and become mindful of the intentions behind our actions and whether they are healthy or harmful. For example, you could be eating a slice of cake because you're enjoying a cup of tea at your favourite café with your sister and they do the best carrot cake. Or, you might be eating cake because your relationship has just ended and cake gives you a temporary distraction from the heartbreak you are unwilling to feel.

Questioning the intentions behind our actions is a fiercely courageous practice that often wakes us up to parts of ourselves that we would usually avoid. Go gently and trust that as you awaken, you will discover a strength and beauty you have hidden from yourself for a very long time. And, as you awaken to this beauty, you will realise you never have to hide again.

Meditation

Soham Meditation

One of the reasons so many of us are disconnected from our true Self is because the world is very loud. We have to deal with so many voices telling us how to behave and what we should do with our lives and who we should be. All this noise in the outside world can make our inner world very noisy too. In order to come home to ourselves, in order to hear the quiet call of our true Self over the roar of our ego and our cultural conditioning and other people's opinions, we have to create an inner silence that draws our awareness inwards.

Mantras help to quieten the mind by filling it with the sound of the mantra instead our usual thoughts, worries and judgements. The mantra *soham*, pronounced 'so'– 'hum', means 'I am that'. It reminds us of our wholeness, that we don't need to cling to identities that are too small for us, that we and the Universe are one.

Begin by finding your meditation posture and allow your mind to settle, using a technique such as Loving Awareness Meditation (*see* p. 101) if you like. Bring your awareness to your breath and begin to silently say 'so' with each inhale and 'hum' with each exhale. As you practise, you might notice that your breathing itself chants *soham* naturally for you and all you need to do is pay attention and listen. This is really what meditation is. An invitation to listen to our true Self. Practise this mantra meditation from five minutes to 20 minutes, or longer if you have time.

Asanas: Backbends

ALLOW ABOUT 50 MINUTES

The way we practise yoga often reflects the way we live our life. Our physical practice often reveals habits and attitudes that are present in the way we eat, the way we work, the way we relate to others and the way we speak to ourselves. As you practise this week, especially as you explore the new backbends, become aware of your habits. Do you have a tendency to strive for the perfect pose? Are you afraid of trying something new? Where is your mind as you practise? What is happening with your breath? Do you rush through your practice, trying to get to the end? Do you skip the poses you find hard? Is your mind ping-ponging all over the place? Are you constantly judging yourself? Our time on the mat allows us to practise *svadhyaya* without the daily distractions of life – phones, emails, chores – so we can begin to untangle the limited idea of who we think we are from the force of love, joy and compassion we have the potential to be.

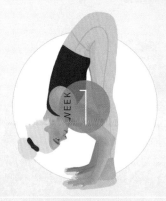

1 **Opening Sequence**
(see p. 58)

2 Repeat WEEK 1:
Standing Forward Bends
(see pp. 86–7)

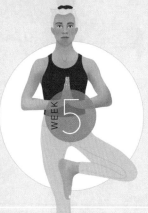

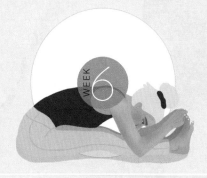

6 Repeat WEEK 5:
Standing Balances
(see pp. 120–1)

7 Repeat WEEK 6:
Seated Forward Bends
(see pp. 130–1)

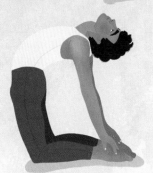

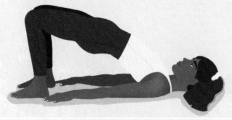

11 **Camel Pose**
(see p. 163), 5 breaths

12 **Bridge Pose**
(see p. 164), 5 breaths

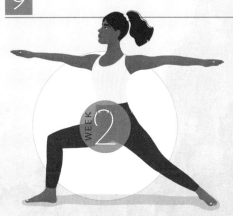

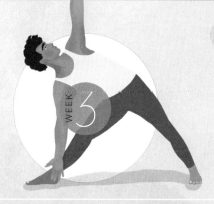

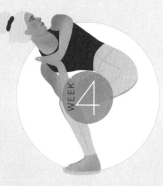

3 Repeat **WEEK 2:**
Leg-strengthening Poses
(*see pp. 94–5*)

4 Repeat **WEEK 3:**
Hip Openers and Hamstring
Stretches (*see pp. 102–3*)

5 Repeat **WEEK 4:**
Revolved Standing Poses
(*see pp. 110–11*)

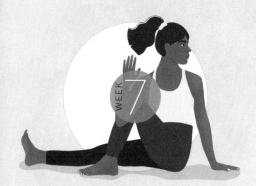

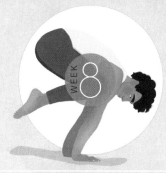

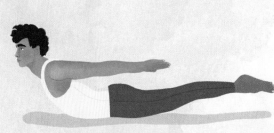

8 Repeat **WEEK 7:**
Seated Twists
(*see pp. 142–3*)

9 Repeat **WEEK 8:**
Arm Balances
(*see pp. 150–1*)

10 **Locust Pose**
(*see p. 162*),
5 breaths

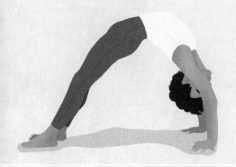

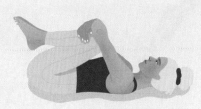

13 **Wheel Pose**
(*see p. 165*) or repeat
Bridge Pose, 5 breaths

14 **Wind-relieving Pose**
(*see p. 166*), 10 breaths

15 **Closing Sequence**
(*see p. 75*)

Locust Pose

SALAMBASANA

This pose strengthens the entire back of the body and prepares us for deeper backbends. Focus on creating length in the pose instead of lift.

1 Lie on your front with your forehead resting on the floor and your feet hip-distance apart. Bring your arms to rest by your sides, palms facing upwards.

2 Reach back through your toes to activate your legs and lengthen through the crown of your head, wrapping your shoulder blades down your back to activate the muscles either side of your spine. Gently push your pubic bone into the floor and draw your navel towards your spine.

3 Inhale, lift your head and peel your upper body off the floor, reaching your breastbone forwards.

4 Lengthen your tailbone towards your heels and reach back through your toes until the tops of your feet begin to float off the floor. If you feel stable here, reach back through your fingers and float your hands off the floor.

5 To exit: Slowly lower yourself back down onto your belly, relaxing the muscles either side of your spine.

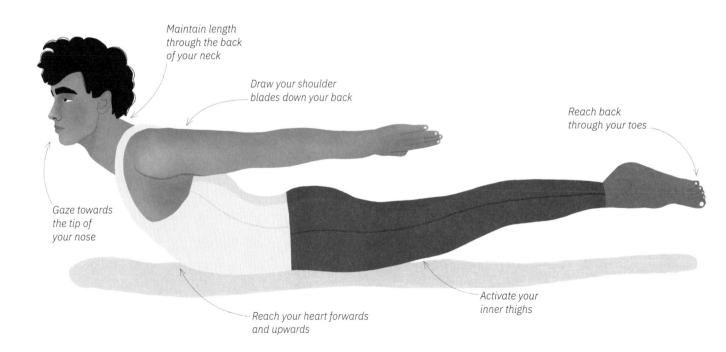

Maintain length through the back of your neck

Draw your shoulder blades down your back

Reach back through your toes

Gaze towards the tip of your nose

Reach your heart forwards and upwards

Activate your inner thighs

Camel Pose

USTRASANA

Camel Pose requires gentleness instead of force. It is a deep backbend and a strong heart opener so give yourself some time to rest afterwards if you need to. Focus on anchoring through your pelvis and opening through your chest.

1 Begin in a high kneeling position with your hips stacked over your knees and your toes either tucked under or pressing the tops of your feet into the mat. Bring your hands to your lower back with your fingers facing downwards.

2 Lengthen your tailbone towards the back of your knees and extend out of your pelvis. Draw your shoulder blades down your back and lift your heart forwards and upwards as you move into the backbend.

3 If you feel stable and are flexible enough, reach for your heels, either keeping your chin tucked or lowering your head back to gaze at the ceiling or the tip of your nose.

4 To exit: Lift your hands to your lower back and, using the strength of your core, lift your torso back to centre.

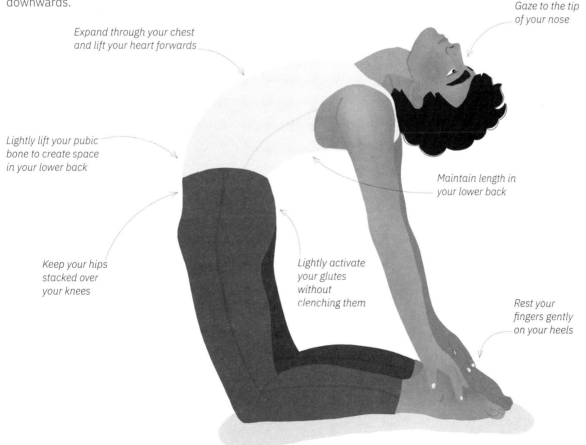

Expand through your chest and lift your heart forwards

Gaze to the tip of your nose

Lightly lift your pubic bone to create space in your lower back

Maintain length in your lower back

Keep your hips stacked over your knees

Lightly activate your glutes without clenching them

Rest your fingers gently on your heels

Bridge Pose

SETU BANDHASANA

This is a gentle backbend and mild inversion. Move into it slowly and mindfully so you can notice the sensations in your body.

1 Lie on your back with your knees bent, feet hip-distance apart, and arms resting by your sides. Make sure the inside edges of your feet are parallel and root downwards through all four corners of each foot.

2 Gently tilt the top front of your pelvis backwards to create length in your lower back and peel your spine off the floor, starting with your tailbone.

3 Press down through your arms, drawing your shoulder blades towards the midline of your body, and lift your chest towards your chin.

4 To exit: Slowly lower down to the ground, starting at the top of your spine, one vertebrae at a time.

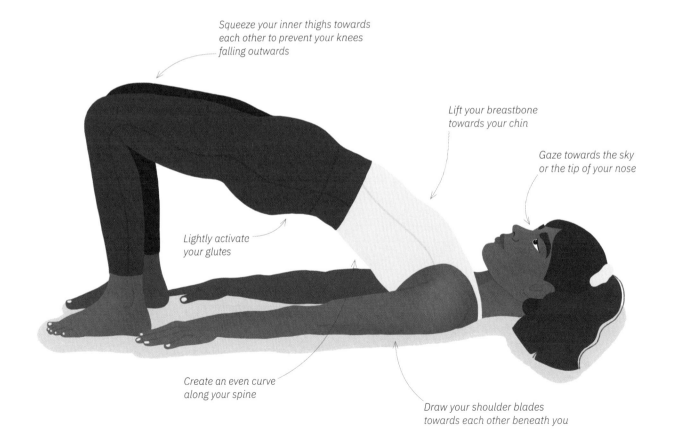

Squeeze your inner thighs towards each other to prevent your knees falling outwards

Lift your breastbone towards your chin

Gaze towards the sky or the tip of your nose

Lightly activate your glutes

Create an even curve along your spine

Draw your shoulder blades towards each other beneath you

Wheel Pose

URDHVA DHANURASANA

This is a deep backbend so listen to your body as you transition into it. If you feel tired or sense a lot of tightness in your body, Bridge Pose (*see* opposite) is a good alternative.

1 Lie on your back with your knees bent, feet hip-distance apart. Make sure the inside edges of your feet are parallel and root downwards through all four corners of each foot. Wrap your elbows in and up to bring your palms to the floor either side of your ears, fingers pointing towards your shoulders.

2 Gently tilt the top front of your pelvis backwards to create length in your lower back. Press your feet and hands firmly into the ground and peel your spine off the floor, starting at your lower spine.

3 As you exhale, push your hands into the floor to lift your head, lowering your crown gently to the mat between your hands. This might be enough for your body so stay here if it is.

4 On your next exhalation, straighten your arms to lift your head off the floor, distributing your weight evenly between your hands and feet, and maintaining an even curve throughout the length of your spine.

5 Press downwards through your hands, drawing your shoulder blades towards the midline of your body, and lift your chest towards your chin.

6 To exit: Tuck your chin towards your chest and lower downwards slowly by bending your arms and legs, lowering from the top of the spine to the tailbone.

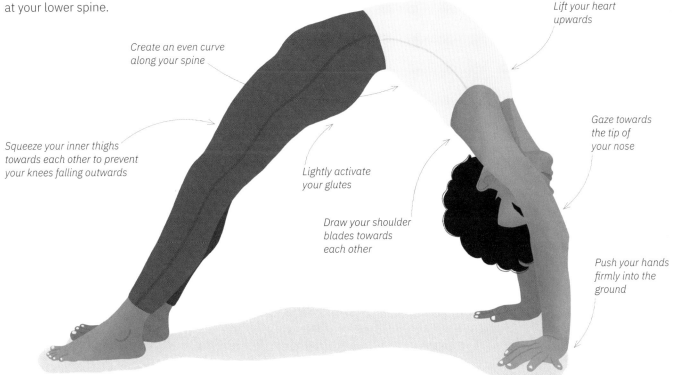

Create an even curve along your spine

Lift your heart upwards

Squeeze your inner thighs towards each other to prevent your knees falling outwards

Gaze towards the tip of your nose

Lightly activate your glutes

Draw your shoulder blades towards each other

Push your hands firmly into the ground

Wind-relieving Pose
PAWANMUKTASANA

This is a comforting counter-pose after a series of backbends. It releases tension in the lower back and can relieve trapped wind from the digestive tract.

1 Lie on your back and hug your knees into your chest, wrapping your arms around your shins.

2 Gently tuck in your chin, close your eyes if you wish, and allow your body to relax into the floor.

3 To exit: Simply release your shins and lengthen your legs out onto the floor.

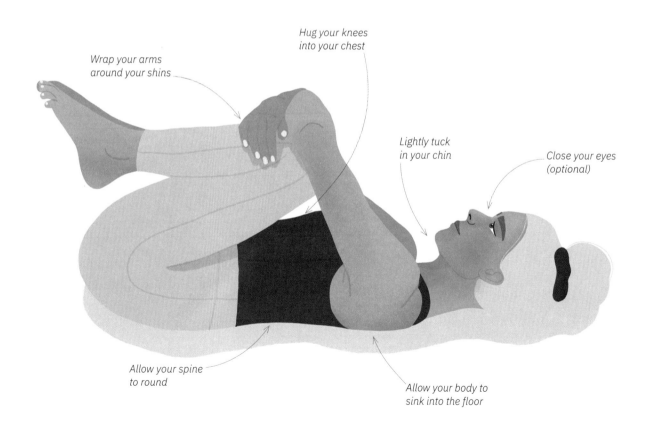

Hug your knees into your chest

Wrap your arms around your shins

Lightly tuck in your chin

Close your eyes (optional)

Allow your spine to round

Allow your body to sink into the floor

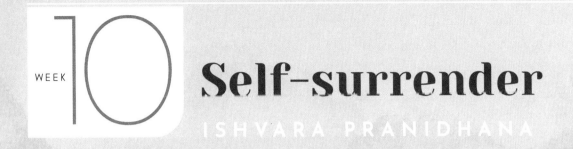

10 Self-surrender

ISHVARA PRANIDHANA

THE FINAL PRACTICE on this ten-week journey is surrender. Letting go. Releasing. This practice of self-surrender – *ishvara pranidhana* – is often the most misunderstood, most resisted and most challenging of all ten pillars of mindful living (*see* p. 22–5). It asks us to release the tight grip we have on life. To let go of control. To have unshakeable faith in the Universe. To walk into the wild unknown. To devote time and energy to nurturing our inner garden, trusting that something beautiful will grow.

In modern, Western culture, we often see surrender as a kind of weakness. Giving up. Quitting. We pride ourselves on having self-control and because having power over our own and other people's lives is promoted as successful, the idea of surrender can feel like failure. In yoga, however, self-surrender is the most powerful thing we can do. By surrendering our ego-desires – for money, fame and control – and the limited idea of who we are (our job, our past, our struggles), we create space for our true Self; for peace, for beauty, for deep, inner joy. Instead of fighting the flow of life, we surrender to it.

The practice of *ishvara pranidhana* cultivates total faith in ourselves and our lives. The word *ishvara* refers to the divine within us, our inner compass, our higher purpose, our limitless capacity for love and compassion. *Pranidhana* means to dedicate, to devote, to trustfully surrender. This act of trustful surrender is not passive. It is not inaction. It does not mean we hand over responsibility for our lives or rely on external spiritual teachers and gurus to tell us how to act and what to believe. Rather, it is the practice of giving ourselves fully to our work, our relationships and our lives without expecting anything in return. It is doing our best and letting go of the outcome. It is working without expecting rewards. It is loving without an agenda. It is having faith that, once we have done all we can do, all that is left is for us to let go and open our hearts. To trust in the Universe. To relax into the flow of life. To know, deep in our hearts, we are exactly where we need to be.

Ishvara pranidhana reminds us to work hard to cultivate the conditions for our healing and transformation and then to let go and let ourselves grow. In this way, yoga is a lot like gardening. We can plant the seeds, we can water them, we can pull out any weeds and protect the seedlings from frost and snow. We can care for them. We can tend to them. But we cannot own them. We cannot control them. We cannot dictate how fast they grow. We cannot force them to bloom. But we can create the optimal conditions and trust that everything blossoms in its own time.

We cannot force ourselves to blossom either. We can't force our hearts to open. We can't force our grief to soften. We can't force ourselves to let go, to heal, to grow. But we can commit to the practices that allow these things to happen: meditation, breathwork, movement, compassion, honesty, gratitude, acceptance, service. Our task here is to trust that within us are the seeds of compassion, wisdom and love and to do the work – both in our inner world and in the outer world – so they can blossom. So *we* can blossom. So, through our blossoming, we can bring a beauty to the world that will inspire others to do the same.

It is only when we wholeheartedly practise self-discipline (*tapas*) and self-study (*svadhyaya*) that we can fully surrender in the knowledge that we have done all we can do. Once we know there is nothing left to do, we can let go. And, as we let go, as we act without selfish motives, as we work in the calm of self-surrender instead of worrying about the outcome, we discover a life force within us that is unstoppable. Because, as we surrender our ego-plans and surface identities, we lose the small, scared, superficial self that keeps us trapped. And, without this 'self', our self-consciousness is transformed to consciousness. The self-consciousness that has haunted us and held us back and left us feeling insecure and unworthy is transformed into pure consciousness; a clear blue sky, unclouded by worry and longing. We are no longer the scared, stressed, self-conscious self, sleepwalking our way through life. We are conscious. Mindful. Present. Aware. Awake. Alive.

Mindful Living Practice

Journal prompts

Oftentimes, we can grasp the idea of self-surrender intellectually but it is much more challenging to actually live in surrender. A good place to start is to practise surrendering any beliefs you have about being unworthy or unloveable, along with any behaviours that these beliefs are being expressed through. Use the questions below to explore where you can practise self-surrender.

What beliefs do I carry about my unworthiness?

What behaviours and habits do I have that express these beliefs?

How would I act differently if I were to surrender these beliefs and reconnect with the divine within me?

What is my personal definition of god or the divine?

Where am I resisting, fighting, or trying to control life?

How can I practise surrender and relax into the flow of life?

Aspiration inspiration

Surrender means saying yes to life instead of fighting against it. Instead of always struggling to paddle upstream, we gently row with the flow. Use the statements below to inspire you to create your own aspirations to remind you to say yes to the present moment and trust in something greater than your ego.

'May I relax into life, knowing that I am exactly where I need to be.'

'May I have trust that by nurturing my inner garden, something beautiful will grow.'

'May I surrender my small, scared self, so I can become more of who I truly am.'

Take a risk and surrender to love

Like any deep transformation, learning to surrender takes time and practice. Beginning by taking tiny risks and practising small moments of surrender will cultivate the trust and faith it takes to fully let go.

Many of us live from a place of fear so surrendering to love, and allowing love to inspire your actions, can be a life-changing practice. This can be love for yourself, for another, or for the whole world.

On a practical level this might look like surrendering to your appetite and feeding yourself from a place of love instead of sticking to a harsh diet because you are afraid your body can't be trusted. For many people, listening to and trusting their body feels risky and vulnerable. Instead of following a strict meal plan, at dinner time ask yourself: 'What would I like to eat right now?' and trust what your body has to say.

Likewise, many of us cram our lives with stuff to do because spending time on our own feels incredibly intimate and vulnerable. If you have a free afternoon, instead of packing it full of chores, ask yourself: 'What would the divine in me like to do right now?' Go for a walk? Clean the house? Light a candle? Read a book? Bake a cake? Have a bath? Journal? Get on my yoga mat? See what happens when you surrender the need to always have a plan or always be productive and simply trust your intuition to guide you.

Another practice is to regularly ask yourself, 'Am I

doing this to earn love or am I doing this from a place of love?' By surrendering the belief that we have to earn love and acting only when we are rooted in love, we move closer to our true Self and our limitless capacity for love.

Breathwork – *pranayama*

Allow your breathwork to be intuitive this week. Ask yourself whether you need a fiery, energising practice like Skull Shining Breath (*see* p. 132) or if the calming, quietening practice of Square Breathing (*see* p. 152) is just what your body and mind are asking for.

Meditation

Meditation techniques are vast and beautiful. In the same way that different types of physical exercise train different aspects of fitness – strength, power, flexibility, cardiovascular health – different types of meditation cultivate different qualities and attitudes, such as presence, awareness, focus, compassion and surrender.

Sometimes the most powerful meditation techniques are the most simple. This week, simplify your meditation practice to just two words: 'let go'. This is particularly transformative for times when your mind is obsessed by compulsive thinking and craving, or when you are fighting against life and resisting reality. Begin to practise it in your formal meditation time – silently saying 'let' as you inhale and 'go' as you exhale – and as you become more comfortable with the technique, introduce it to those anxious moments in daily life when you notice yourself trying to control the uncontrollable. Again, practise for anywhere from five minutes to 20 minutes, noticing when there is resistance to practising and how you feel after you do.

Reminding ourselves to let go again and again empowers us to deal with the unpredictability of life in a more balanced way. To open our hearts to whatever the Universe gifts us. To let go of the desire to have everything neat, ordered and under control, and instead fall in love with the whole sacred messiness of life.

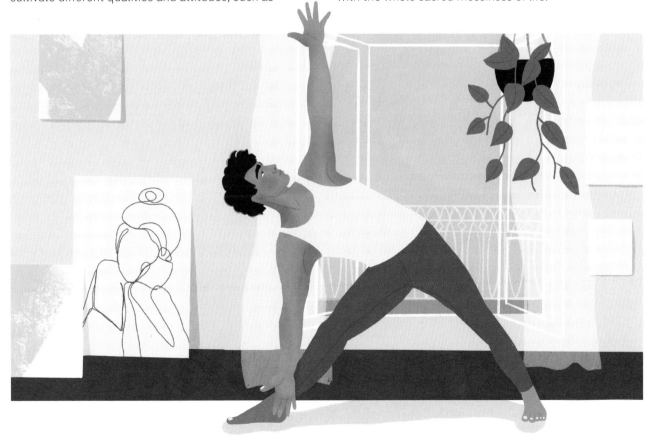

Asanas: Soothing Yin Poses

ALLOW ABOUT 60 MINUTES

Surrender is an act of strength. It takes a gentle courage to release our idea of what our self-practice should look like, how much our body should weigh, how our partner should behave or how our life should be, and instead to surrender to each moment exactly as it is. Time on the mat gives us the opportunity to practise and experience self-surrender, especially in the soothing yin poses that are the final addition to our sequence. This week, see how it feels to devote your practice to someone other than yourself. Treat each forward bend as a bow of respect and gratitude and each backbend as a way to open your heart to love and to offer this love to the Universe. If your body is asking for something different this week, trust it. There are more sequences to explore in Part Three of the book (*see* p. 176).

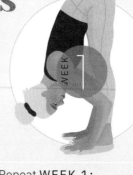

1 **Opening Sequence** (*see p. 58*)

2 Repeat **WEEK 1:** **Standing Forward Bends** (*see pp. 86–7*)

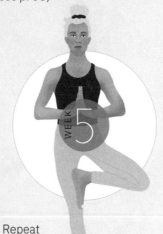

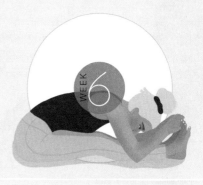

6 Repeat **WEEK 5:** **Standing Balances** (*see pp. 120–1*)

7 Repeat **WEEK 6:** **Seated Forward Bends** (*see pp. 130–1*)

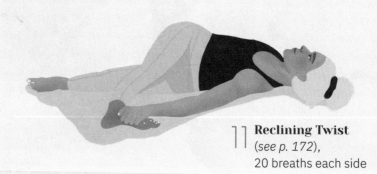

11 **Reclining Twist** (*see p. 172*), 20 breaths each side

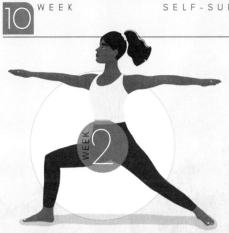

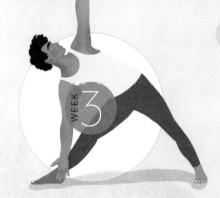

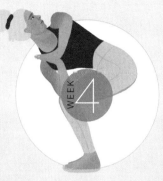

3 Repeat **WEEK 2:**
Leg-strengthening Poses
(*see pp. 94–5*)

4 Repeat **WEEK 3:**
**Hip Openers and
Hamstring Stretches**
(*see pp. 102–3*)

5 Repeat **WEEK 4:**
Revolved Standing Poses
(*see pp. 110–11*)

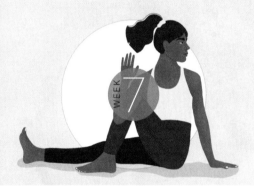

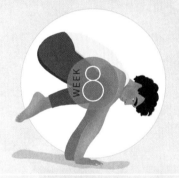

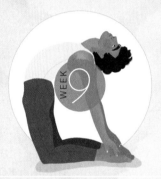

8 Repeat **WEEK 7:**
Seated Twists
(*see pp. 142–3*)

9 Repeat **WEEK 8:**
Arm Balances
(*see pp. 150–1*)

10 Repeat **WEEK 9:**
Backbends
(*see pp. 160–1*)

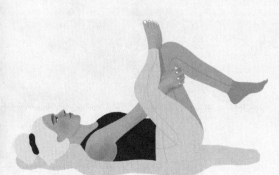

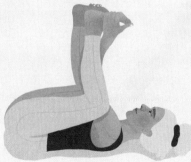

12 **Reclining Pigeon Pose**
(*see p. 173*),
20 breaths each side

13 **Happy Baby Pose**
(*see p. 174*),
20 breaths

14 **Closing Sequence**
(*see p. 75*)

Reclining Twist

SUPTA MATSYENDRASANA

This is a calming twist that relieves tension from the spine and brings balance to the body after a dynamic practice. Focus on softening into this pose rather than actively stretching.

1 Lie on your back and hug your right knee into your chest.

2 Take hold of the outside of your right foot or knee with your left hand and guide your right leg across your body. Keep the knee bent for a gentler twist or straighten it if you want a slightly deeper stretch.

3 Keeping both shoulder blades on the floor, reach your right arm out to the right side and gaze over your right shoulder or upwards to the sky.

4 To exit: Draw your right leg back to centre, before repeating on the other side.

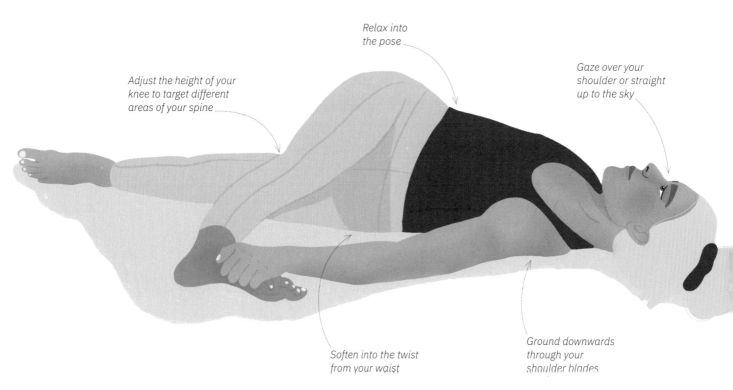

Relax into the pose

Gaze over your shoulder or straight up to the sky

Adjust the height of your knee to target different areas of your spine

Soften into the twist from your waist

Ground downwards through your shoulder blades

Reclining Pigeon Pose

SUPTA EKA PADA GALAVASANA

This pose releases tension from the lower back and hips. Work with your body gently in this pose, focusing on softening and opening.

1 Lie on your back with your knees bent and feet flat on the floor. Lift your right leg and place your right ankle across your right thigh, allowing your right hip to open. Flex your right foot to protect your knee.

2 Thread your right hand through the space between your legs and reach your left hand around the outside of your left thigh, clasping your hands behind your left thigh and drawing your leg towards you.

3 Keep your shoulders grounded and relax your tailbone towards the floor, allowing the muscles around your hip to soften.

4 To exit: Release your right foot back to the floor and repeat on the other side.

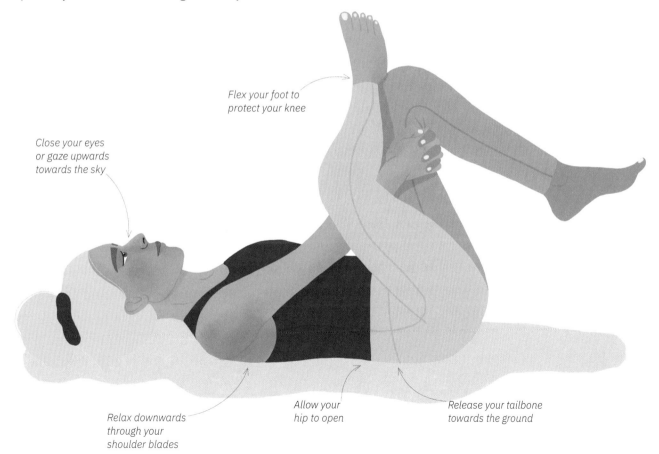

Flex your foot to protect your knee

Close your eyes or gaze upwards towards the sky

Relax downwards through your shoulder blades

Allow your hip to open

Release your tailbone towards the ground

Happy Baby Pose

ANADA BALASANA

This is a beautiful, restorative pose. Feel free to go straight to Corpse Pose (*see* p. 81) afterwards.

1 Lie on your back and draw your knees towards your armpits, taking hold of the outside edges of your feet.

2 Allow your legs to open wide and your knees to sink down towards the floor.

3 Either relax here or rock gently from side to side to massage your spine.

4 To exit: Release your big toes and lengthen out your legs, relaxing into the floor.

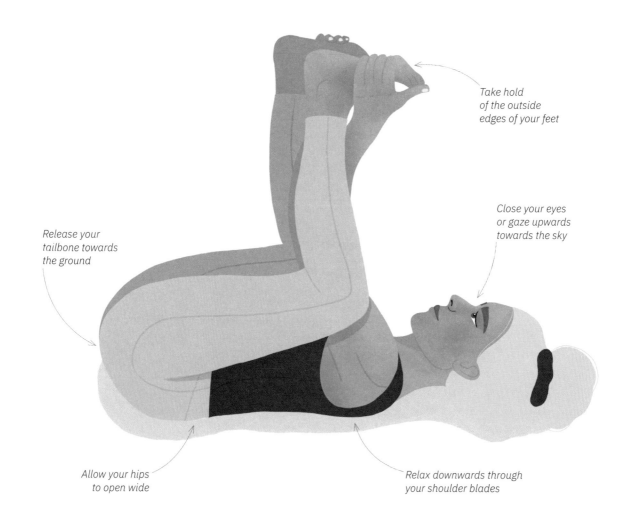

Take hold of the outside edges of your feet

Close your eyes or gaze upwards towards the sky

Release your tailbone towards the ground

Allow your hips to open wide

Relax downwards through your shoulder blades

Where now?

My hope for you is that you have discovered that the practice of yoga is a portal to an inner universe. A spiritual journey back home to your own body, your own breath, your own Earth. A sacred space where you can find your Self over and over again.

I hope that yoga has felt like turning on a light. That it has opened your eyes to a different way of seeing yourself and the world. That it has given you the capacity to go to the dark places you have spent a lifetime running from and to discover the gifts that hide there.

I hope you are beginning to embrace all parts of yourself. The beauty. The regret. The grief. The dreams. The shame-filled parts hiding in the dark and dusty corners of your soul. The nooks and crannies that are calling out to be seen.

I hope that you are beginning to trust yourself and your inner wisdom and the quiet call of your heart. That you are fully inhabiting your own skin instead of being ashamed of it. That you are treating this little part of the Universe as sacred.

I hope you are discovering that yoga is a certain way of being alive. An intensification of life. A completeness. A fullness. A wholeness. A celebration of your connection to a greater power that is grounded in deep love and compassion for your Self and for all beings.

As we come to the end of this journey, I hope you continue. I hope you continue to return to your yoga mat, your meditation cushion, your journal. I hope you continue to weave yoga into your daily life through your love and tenderness and tiny humble acts of kindness. I hope you continue healing and growing and transforming your suffering into something sacred, because the lessons we learn from our suffering can become a gift for the world. I hope you continue to become more of who you are.

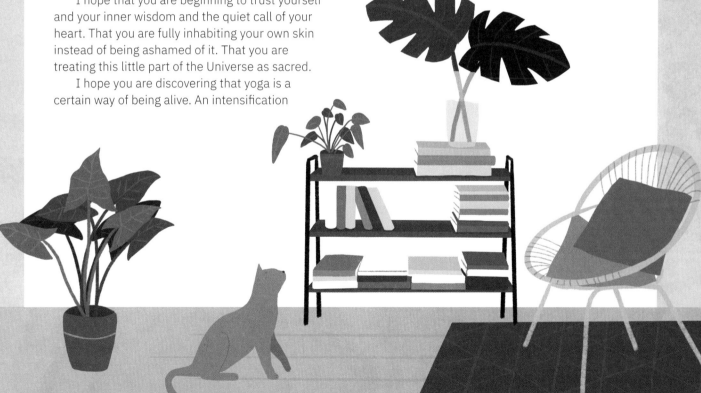

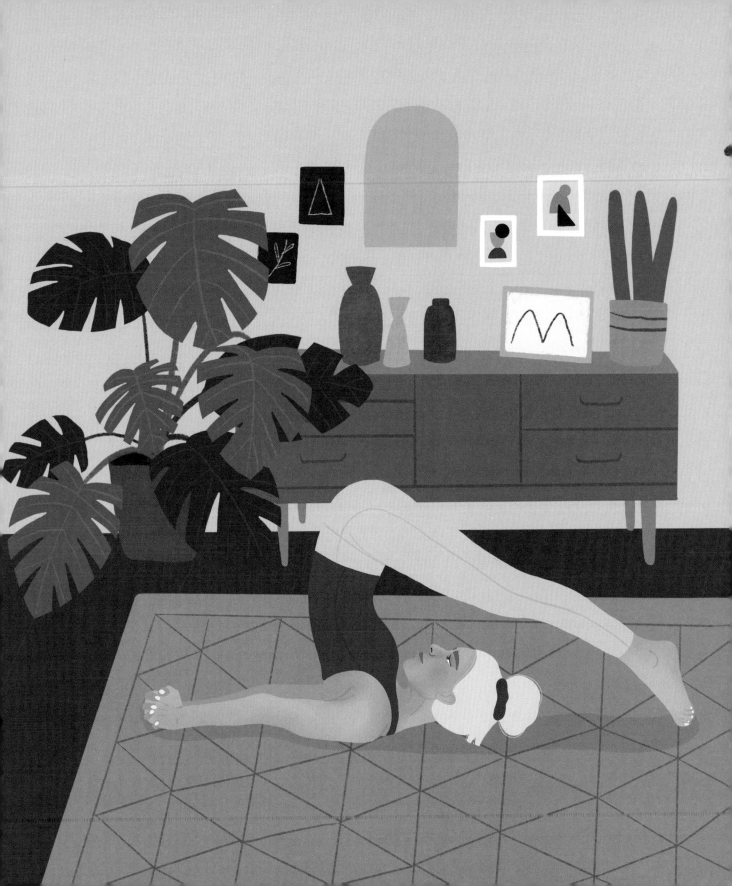

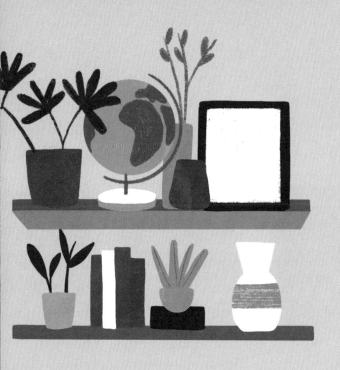

PART THREE
Explore

As you move through the ten-week journey, you may notice there are days when your body needs something different: something calmer, slower, more opening, more soothing. Each time you step on your mat, ask your body what it needs and then be patient enough to listen to what it has to say. Explore the sequences in this section to help you answer it. Each one takes only ten to 15 minutes so is perfect for when you have time for only a short practice.

Grounding

Stay centred with this
sequence of strong, dynamic
poses. It is perfect for those
busy days when you're
feeling out of balance.

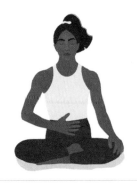

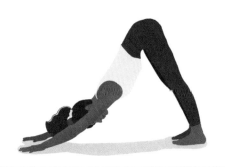

1 **Equal Breathing**
(*see p. 62*), 2 minutes

2 **Downward Dog**
(*see p. 72*), 10 breaths

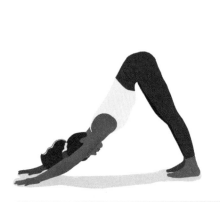

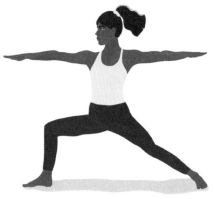

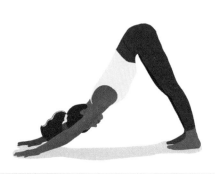

6 **Downward Dog**,
10 breaths

7 **Warrior Two**,
right leg forwards, 10 breaths

8 **Downward Dog**,
10 breaths

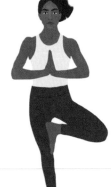

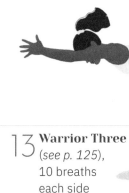

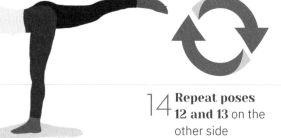

12 **Tree Pose**
(*see p. 122*),
10 breaths then
transition to
next pose

13 **Warrior Three**
(*see p. 125*),
10 breaths
each side

14 **Repeat poses
12 and 13** on the
other side

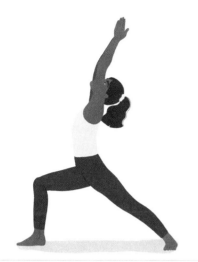

3 **Warrior One,**
right leg forwards (*see p. 74*),
10 breaths

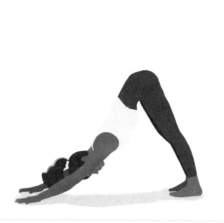

4 **Downward Dog,**
10 breaths

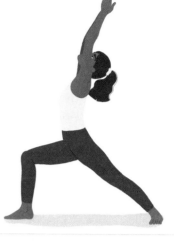

5 **Warrior One,**
left leg forwards, 10 breaths

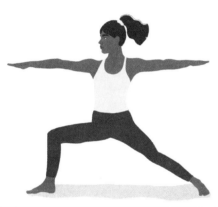

9 **Warrior Two,**
left leg forwards,
10 breaths

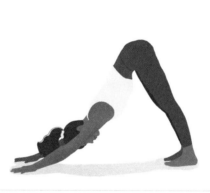

10 **Downward Dog,**
10 breaths

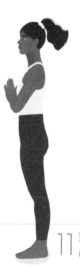

11 **Mountain Pose**
(*see p. 64*), 10 breaths

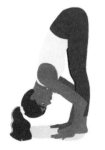

15 **Standing
Forward Bend**
(*see p. 66*),
10 breaths

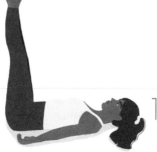

16 **Legs Up the Wall
Pose** (*see p. 79*),
2 minutes

17 **Corpse Pose**
(*see p. 81*), 5–10
minutes

Releasing

Let go of physical and emotional tension with this sequence of hip and heart openers.

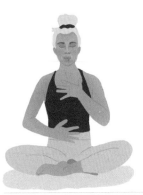

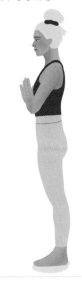

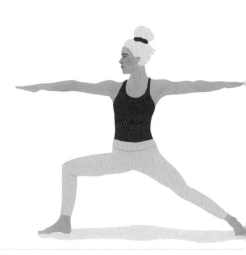

1 **Square Breathing**
(*see p. 152*), 2 minutes

2 **Mountain Pose**
(*see p. 64*), 5 breaths

3 **Warrior Two**
(*see p. 97*), 5 breaths
then transition to next pose

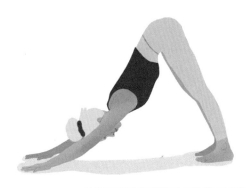

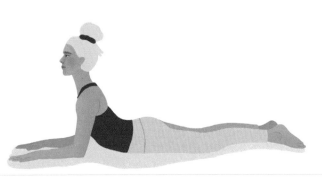

7 **Downward Dog**
(*see p. 72*)

8 **Cobra Pose**
(*see p. 71*), 5 breaths

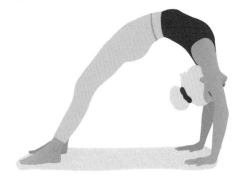

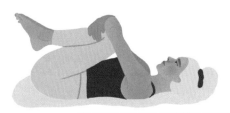

12 **Wheel Pose**
(*see p. 165*) or repeat Bridge Pose, 5 breaths

13 **Wind-relieving Pose**
(*see p. 166*), 5 breaths

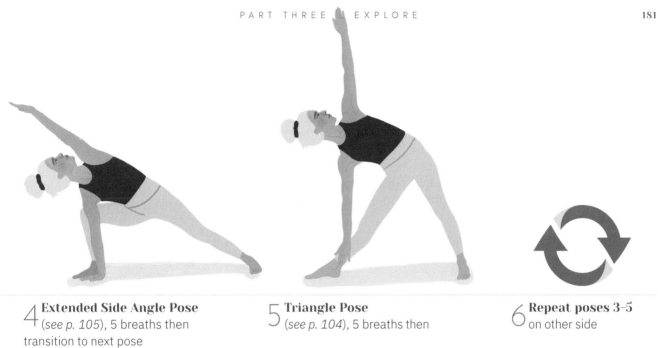

4 **Extended Side Angle Pose**
(*see p. 105*), 5 breaths then
transition to next pose

5 **Triangle Pose**
(*see p. 104*), 5 breaths then

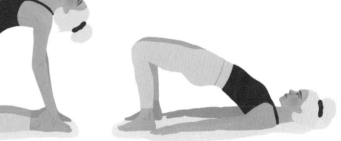

6 **Repeat poses 3–5**
on other side

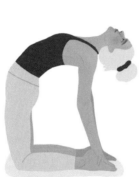

9 **Upward Dog**
(*see p. 70*), 5 breaths

10 **Camel Pose**
(*see p. 163*), 5 breaths

11 **Bridge Pose**
(*see p. 164*), 5 breaths

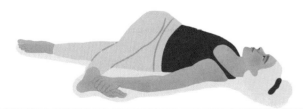

14 **Reclining Twist**
(*see p. 172*), 2 minutes each side

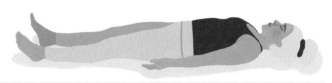

15 **Corpse Pose**
(*see p. 81*), 5–10 minutes

Energising

A powerful sequence to boost energy, uplift and rejuvenate.

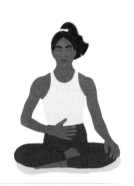

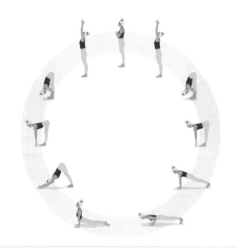

1 **Skull Shining Breath**
(*see p. 132*), 5 rounds

2 **Sun Salutation A**
(*see p.59*), 3 rounds

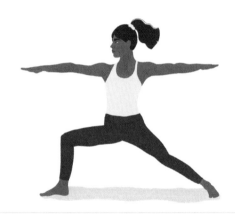

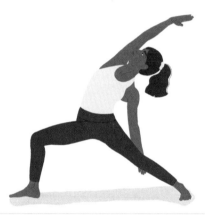

6 **Warrior Two**
(*see p. 97*), 5 breaths then transition to next pose

7 **Reverse Warrior**
(*see p. 98*), 5 breaths then transition to next pose

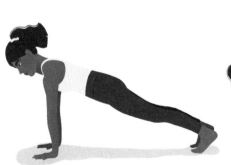

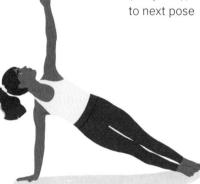

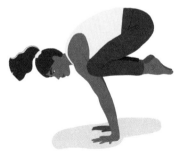

11 **Plank Pose**
(*see p. 68*), 10 breaths

12 **Side Plank Pose**
(*see p. 153*), 5 breaths

13 **Crow Pose**
(*see p. 154*), play with this for 1–2 minutes

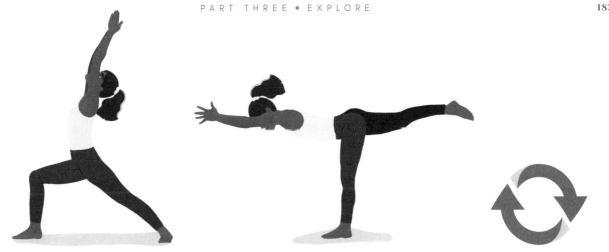

3 **Warrior One**
(*see p. 74*), 5 breaths then transition to next pose

4 **Warrior Three**
(*see p. 125*), 5 breaths

5 **Repeat poses 3 and 4**
on other side

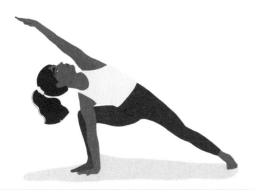
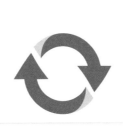
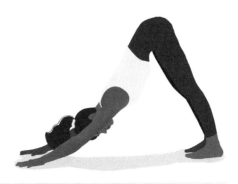

8 **Extended Side Angle Pose**
(*see p. 105*), 5 breaths then transition

9 **Repeat poses 6–8**
on the other side

10 **Sun Salutation A,**
1 round ending in Downward Dog

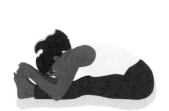
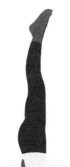
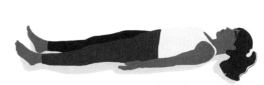
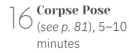

14 **Seated Forward Bend**
(*see p. 134*), 10 breaths

15 **Shoulder Stand**
(*see p. 77*), 10 breaths

16 **Corpse Pose**
(*see p. 81*), 5–10 minutes

Calming

A slow and gentle evening routine that calms the nervous system so you can sleep well.

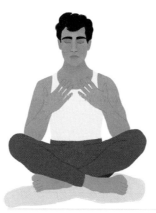

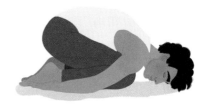

1 **Three-part Breath**
(*see p. 112*), 2 minutes

2 **Child's Pose**
(*see p. 156*), 2 minutes

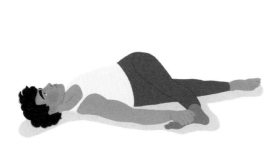

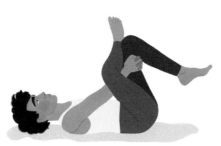

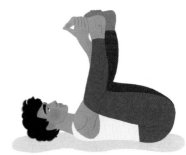

3 **Reclining Twist**
(*see p. 172*), 2 minutes each side

4 **Reclining Pigeon Pose**
(*see p. 173*), 2 minutes each side

5 **Happy Baby Pose**
(*see p. 174*), 2 minutes

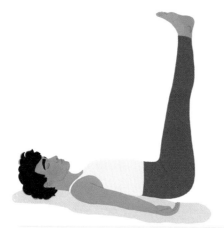

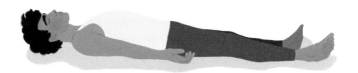

6 **Legs Up the Wall Pose**
(*see p. 79*), 2 minutes

7 **Corpse Pose**
(*see p. 81*), 5–10 minutes

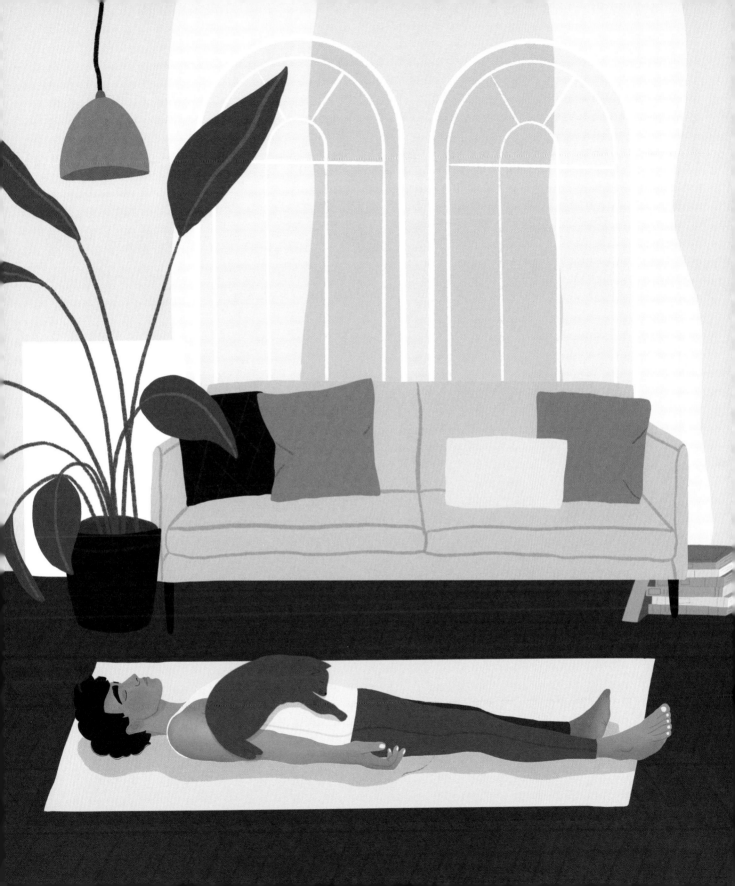

References

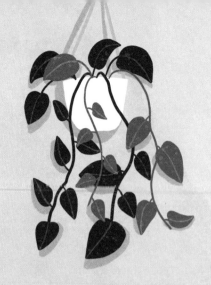

THE FIVE BRANCHES OF HEALTH

Dagar, C., Pandey, A., Navare, A. V. & Pandey, N. (2018, July). How Yoga Based Practices Result in Human Flourishing?. In *Academy of Management Proceedings* (Vol. 2018, No. 1, p. 16300). Briarcliff Manor, NY 10510: Academy of Management

Dhar, N., Chaturvedi, S. K. & Nandan, D. (2011). Spiritual health scale 2011: Defining and measuring 4th dimension of health. *Indian Journal of Community Medicine: official publication of Indian Association of Preventive & Social Medicine*, 36(4), 275

Grossman, P. (2015). Mindfulness: awareness informed by an embodied ethic. *Mindfulness*, 6(1), 17–22

Holt-Lunstad, J., Smith, T. B., Baker, M., Harris, T. & Stephenson, D. (2015). Loneliness and social isolation as risk factors for mortality: a meta-analytic review. *Perspectives on psychological science*, 10(2), 227–237

Jordan, M. & Hinds, J. (2016). *Ecotherapy: Theory, research and practice*. Macmillan International Higher Education

Musial, J. (2016). Body Vigilance and Orthorexia in Yoga Spaces. *Yoga, the body, and embodied social change: An intersectional feminist analysis*, 141

Pietromonaco, P. R. & Collins, N. L. (2017). Interpersonal mechanisms linking close relationships to health. *American Psychologist*, 72(6), 531

Ross, A. & Thomas, S. (2010). The health benefits of yoga and exercise: a review of comparison studies. *The journal of alternative and complementary medicine*, 16(1), 3–12

Taneja, D. K. (2014). Yoga and health. *Indian Journal of Community Medicine: official publication of Indian Association of Preventive & Social Medicine*, 39(2), 68.
Vader, J. P. (2006). Spiritual health: the next frontier

THE UNIVERSE OF THE BODY

Delaney, K. & Anthis, K. (2010). Is women's participation in different types of yoga classes associated with different levels of body awareness satisfaction?. *International Journal of Yoga Therapy*, 20(1), 62–71

Mental Health Foundation (2019). Body image: how we think and feel about our bodies. *Retrieved from* www.mentalhealth.org.uk

THE JOURNEY

Brown, R. P. & Gerbarg, P. L. (2005). Sudarshan Kriya Yogic breathing in the treatment of stress, anxiety, and depression: part II – clinical applications and guidelines. *Journal of Alternative & Complementary Medicine*, 11(4), 711–717

Colzato, L. S., Barone, H., Sellaro, R. & Hommel, B. (2017). More attentional focusing through binaural beats: evidence from the global–local task. *Psychological research*, 81(1), 271–277

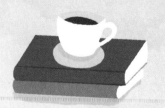

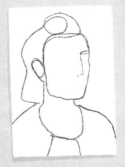

Fisher, J. P., Young, C. N., & Fadel, P. J. (2009). Central sympathetic overactivity: maladies and mechanisms. *Autonomic Neuroscience*, 148(1–2), 5–15

Jerath, R., Edry, J. W., Barnes, V. A. & Jerath, V. (2006). Physiology of long pranayamic breathing: neural respiratory elements may provide a mechanism that explains how slow deep breathing shifts the autonomic nervous system. *Medical hypotheses*, 67(3), 566–571

Sharma, V. K., Rajajeyakumar, M., Velkumary, S., Subramanian, S. K., Bhavanani, A. B., Madanmohan, A. S. & Thangavel, D. (2014). Effect of fast and slow *pranayama* practice on cognitive functions in healthy volunteers. *Journal of Clinical and Diagnostic Research: JCDR*, 8(1), 10

Sharma, V. K., Trakroo, M., Subramaniam, V., Rajajeyakumar, M., Bhavanani, A. B. & Sahai, A. (2013). Effect of fast and slow *pranayama* on perceived stress and cardiovascular parameters in young health-care students. *International Journal of Yoga*, 6(2), 104

SELF-CARE TO ENHANCE YOUR PRACTICE

Aviva (2017) Sleepless cities revealed as one in three adults suffer from insomnia. *Retrieved from* www.aviva.com

Krause, A. J., Simon, E. B., Mander, B. A., Greer, S. M., Saletin, J. M., Goldstein-Piekarski, A. N. & Walker, M. P. (2017). The sleep-deprived human brain. *Nature Reviews Neuroscience*, 18(7), 404

Pearce, M. J., Smigelsky, M. A. & Neimeyer, R. A. (2015). Spiritual journaling. *Techniques of grief therapy: Assessment and intervention*, 205–208

Smyth, J. M., Hockemeyer, J. R. & Tulloch, H. (2008). Expressive writing and post-traumatic stress disorder: Effects on trauma symptoms, mood states, and cortisol reactivity. *British Journal of Health Psychology*, 13(1), 85–93

Walker, M. (2017). *Why We Sleep: Unlocking the Power of Sleep and Dreams*. London: Simon and Schuster

Williams, G. B., Gerardi, M. B., Gill, S. L., Soucy, M. D. & Taliaferro, D. H. (2009). Reflective journaling: Innovative strategy for self-awareness for graduate nursing students. *International Journal of Human Caring*, 13(3), 36–43

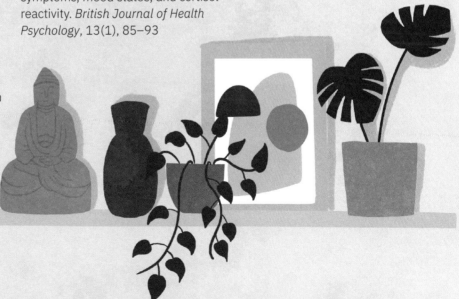

Recommended Reading

This book would not have been possible without the inspiration and wisdom of numerous devoted teachers, authors, researchers, psychotherapists and practitioners, many of whom I came across via their books. I have included a selection of these books below as well as some traditional scripture to inspire you on your journey.

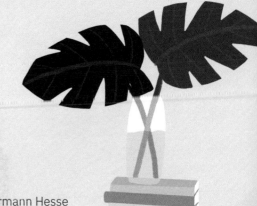

A New Earth: Awakening To Your Life's Purpose by Eckhart Tolle

A Path With Heart: The Classic Guide Through the Perils and Promises of Spiritual Life by Jack Kornfield

A Pukka Life: Finding Your Path to Perfect Health by Sebastian Cole

Autobiography of a Yogi by Paramahansa Yogananda

Ayurveda: The Science of Self-healing by Vasant Lad

Be Here Now by Ram Dass

Change Your Thoughts, Change Your Life: Living the Wisdom of the Tao by Wayne Dyer

Daring Greatly: How the Courage to Be Vulnerable Changes the Way We Live, Love, Parent and Lead by Brene Brown

Falling Upward: A Spirituality For the Two Halves of Life by Richard Rohr

Freedom From the Known by Jiddu Krishnamurti

I Am That by Sri Nisargadatta Maharaj

If Woman Rose Rooted: The Journey to Authenticity and Belonging by Sharon Blackie

In the Realm of Hungry Ghosts by Gabor Maté

Radical Acceptance: Embracing Your Life With the Heart of a Buddha by Tara Brach

Real Love: The Art of Mindful Connection by Sharon Salzberg

Siddhartha by Hermann Hesse

Tao Te Ching by Lao Tzu

The Artist's Way: A Spiritual Path to Higher Creativity by Julia Cameron

The Bhagavad Gita translated by Eknath Easwaran

The Dhammapada translated by Eknath Easwaran

The Four Noble Truths of Love: Buddhist Wisdom For Modern Relationships by Susan Piver

The More Beautiful World Our Hearts Know is Possible by Charles Eisenstein

The Places That Scare You: A Guide to Fearlessness by Pema Chödrön

The Seven Spiritual Laws of Yoga by Deepak Chopra

The Untethered Soul by Michael Singer

The Upanishads translated by Eknath Easwaran

Touching Enlightenment: Finding Realization in the Body by Reginald Ray

Yoga Sutras of Pantanjali translated by Sri Swami Satchidananda

Why Buddhism is True: The Science And Philosophy of Meditation and Enlightenment by Robert Wright

Women Who Run with the Wolves by Clarissa Pinkola Estes

Index

Acknowledgements

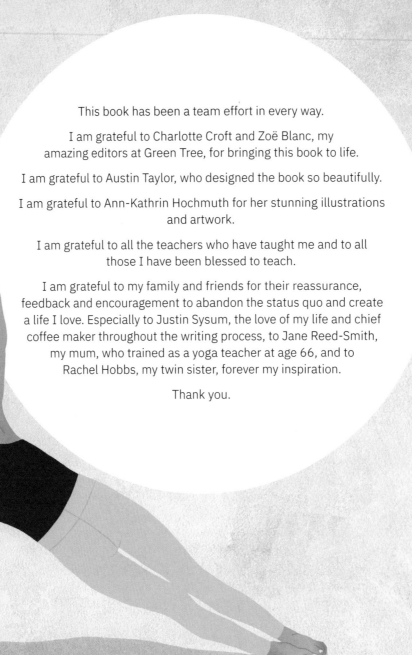

This book has been a team effort in every way.

I am grateful to Charlotte Croft and Zoë Blanc, my amazing editors at Green Tree, for bringing this book to life.

I am grateful to Austin Taylor, who designed the book so beautifully.

I am grateful to Ann-Kathrin Hochmuth for her stunning illustrations and artwork.

I am grateful to all the teachers who have taught me and to all those I have been blessed to teach.

I am grateful to my family and friends for their reassurance, feedback and encouragement to abandon the status quo and create a life I love. Especially to Justin Sysum, the love of my life and chief coffee maker throughout the writing process, to Jane Reed-Smith, my mum, who trained as a yoga teacher at age 66, and to Rachel Hobbs, my twin sister, forever my inspiration.

Thank you.